Tennis Injury Handbook

Professional Advice for Amateur Athletes

Allan M. Levy, M.D.
Mark L. Fuerst

John Wiley & Sons, Inc.

New York • Chichester • Weinheim • Brisbane • Singapore • Toronto

Library of Congress Cataloging-in-Publication Data:

Levy, Allan M.
    Tennis injury handbook : professional advice for amateur athletes /
  Allan M. Levy & Mark L. Fuerst.
       p.   cm.
    Includes index.
    ISBN 0-471-24854-1
    1. Tennis injuries—Handbooks, manuals, etc.   I. Fuerst, Mark.
  II. Title.
  RC1220.T4L49   1999
  617.1′027—dc21   98-33165

Printed in the United States of America

10 9 8 7 6 5 4 3 2 1

Contents

Exercises

Foreword

Physical conditioning and stretching are fundamental to playing good tennis. Almost all of today's top players follow detailed training programs and have their own personal trainers. Many tennis players of all levels who attend my tennis development courses want advice on flexibility and strength training. They have become aware that without good range of motion and power, they can't hit the ball the way they want to.

In *Tennis Injury Handbook,* you will get great information from Dr. Allan Levy and Mark Fuerst. These two top professionals can give you the latest, cutting-edge information on sports medicine. I'm sure that if you follow their advice, you will be able to do more with the tennis racquet and reach your full tennis potential. And you'll have much more fun playing the game.

This book will help you prepare for a wide variety of potential problems. It includes advice and ideas on preventing injuries before they happen, as well as fixing temporary physical problems that may develop if you play tennis on a regular basis.

In short, this book will help you get ready to play the best tennis of your life.

—Dennis Van der Meer
President and founder of the
Van der Meer Tennis University
and of the United States
Professional Tennis Registry

Acknowledgments

We would like to thank the many people who helped make this book possible. John "Mother" Dunn, strength coach of the New York football Giants, for his suggestions with the conditioning and strength programs; John Mancuso, video director of the Giants, for his help in putting the exercise illustrations together; Stuart Holland, private trainer nonpareil, for suggesting and providing access to various exercises; our agent, Faith Hamlin, of Sanford J. Greenburger Associates, Inc., for continuing to guide us in spreading the word; Judith McCarthy and the staff at John Wiley for editorial and production quality; Jackie Aher for her skillful illustrations; and John B. Harris, a good friend, for his avid support and consummate contacts.

To my wife, Gail, who not only put up with my extra hours putting this down on paper, but then did all of my typing, copying, and faxing as well.—AML

To my wife, Margie, for her continued support and patience during my long nights of writing and editing the manuscript. To Ben, for reminding me how much fun it is to get out, run around, and hit balls with a tennis racquet.—MLF

Introduction

What makes a great tennis player? You definitely have to be in shape. You also have to be strong, have real agility, be able to react quickly, and have good explosion to the ball. And then you have to have recovery. When you're pushed out wide, you have to be able to get back.

You don't necessarily have to be born with the proper body, but you do have to use that body properly. If you work diligently, you can add more foot speed and a reliable volley to your repertoire and be able to pound in your serve.

The good thing about tennis is that almost everyone can play it. You can play tennis for sport, for recreation, and even for the exercise benefits it provides. You can play it outdoors in good weather, or indoors in bad weather. You can play singles or doubles. You can play for the fun of it or you can play it competitively. You can also play it at any skill level, from novice to tournament expert.

And you can get some important physical benefits from the sport. You can improve your heart pumping activity, gain muscle tone, and improve blood circulation to your legs (particularly if you are older and play on a regular basis). A half hour of tennis singles against a similarly skilled opponent three times a week can improve your health and endurance.

One of the more attractive elements of tennis is its relatively low rate of injury. Nevertheless, some players do get hurt while playing, and this can detract from both the pleasure and the performance of the game.

Because tennis is played at many levels, different types of injury occur. When you compare an athletic 20-year-old college student playing singles with a 65-year-old playing doubles, you realize just how varied the game can be. Although intensity places the young, competitive athlete at a greater risk for injury than the older, less competitive player, the greater strength and flexibility of youth may help protect against some of the stresses and strains of the game.

My major concern in managing acute tennis injuries is to prevent them from becoming chronic. Once they become chronic, you can incur long-term disability and decrease your playing time. My tennis playing patients may clamor to get back onto the court, but I make certain they don't return prematurely.

The majority of tennis injuries are due to overuse. Many can be traced to improper technique, and most can be self-treated or treated by a doctor successfully. The treatment and rehabilitation of typical tennis injuries such as ankle sprains, Achilles tendinitis, muscle strains, tennis elbow, rotator cuff problems, cartilage tears, and plantar fasciitis varies from rest and an exercise program to minor surgery. In addition to medical treatment and rehabilitation, alterations in tennis equipment and technique can speed a player's recovery.

This book will show you some of the best sport-specific training moves for tennis. Make the moves a regular part of your fitness regimen. After just a few sessions, you'll find that you move more confidently during play. Devote a month or more, and you'll gain strength and flexibility that will help you put your skills to use and avoid injury. Sport-specific training won't turn you into a tennis pro overnight. But I guarantee it will boost your performance.

HOW TO USE THIS BOOK

In Part One, I take you through the essential elements of a proper workout to improve your game. That includes warm-up and stretching, conditioning, and strength training. I also provide sound advice on what foods to eat before, during, and after a match for peak performance.

The stretching program will increase your flexibility. Flexibility is particularly important for the middle-aged tennis player who tries to swing a racquet the first nice spring weekend. Returning to action after a long layoff puts you at high risk of an injury. Overstretching a joint or muscle may result in a sprain or muscle pull, causing many miserable Mondays after a weekend of tennis.

The strength-training program will help you build muscles throughout the body. All tennis players would like to hit the fuzz off the ball and overpower their opponents, and strength training can help you do that without compromising flexibility.

In Part Two, I focus on common concerns and fundamental precautions for tennis players regarding who gets injured, and medical problems they may face. I also review tennis gadgets being marketed to enhance your health and to improve strength and flexibility.

Part Three provides a complete guide to tennis injuries, organized by area of the body, from head to toe. You will learn how to recognize and treat injuries to each body part and determine when it's safe to play again. You'll also discover how to prevent reinjury using specific exercises. I give practical advice, not just theoretical applications. For example, to strengthen your wrists, you can squeeze a soft rubber ball bought from a five-and-dime store.

I also note when an amateur's injury is different from a professional's. A weekend tennis player with a sore shoulder may have stretched out the rotator cuff muscles across the top of the shoulder, and for these athletes, simple exercises usually reduce the stress on the shoulder joint. Only a professional tennis player is likely to need surgery for a rotator cuff problem.

Any amateur can learn the rehabilitation techniques that professional tennis players use. Weekend warriors may not have the time to devote to rehabilitating themselves and working on their games as pros do, but the methods are the same. It's just a matter of degree.

Next to each condition in Part Three you'll find a symbol. These symbols help you understand whether you can begin to self-treat the condition or whether you must see a doctor or go for emergency treatment. The conditions are coded in the following way:

The first-aid symbol indicates that you may be able to treat the condition on your own initially with some basic first aid, though you may have to see a doctor later. Most tennis injuries fall into this category—for example, a sprained ankle from stepping on a ball on the court.

This symbol means that you need to see a doctor directly for treatment, even though the injury may seem to be minor and not that painful, such as pain at the base of your hand. While you may have only bruised your hand, it's possible you may have broken a small bone and will need to see a doctor to get an X ray.

EMERGENCY

This symbol indicates an emergency situation—a condition such as tearing up a knee from a sudden directional change that needs immediate medical treatment in a hospital or emergency care facility.

Part Four offers additional information on special concerns for female, senior, and young tennis players, including special tips on how they can improve their games.

Part One

Preparing to Play

Work Out to Win
Eat to Compete

1

Work Out to Win

I know it's tempting to just go out and play tennis, or to rush through the time you spend preparing to play. But when you don't work out properly, you risk muscle soreness, decreased performance, and injury.

If you play tennis regularly, you probably need a workout master plan. That's what this chapter offers you. The plan can be summarized in six simple steps:

1. Warm up properly.
2. Take time to stretch.
3. Include agility and speed training.
4. Add in conditioning or strengthening exercises.
5. Warm down gradually.
6. Stretch again.

You may be surprised to learn how many injuries can be prevented by following these steps. You may be familiar with some of this information, but as you read carefully and begin to incorporate it into your tennis game, you will discover the difference it makes. This information is the basis for minimizing strains, sprains, tears, and other hidden hazards.

A physically fit tennis player is more likely to be a successful tennis player. The goal of the workout plan is to help you become a stronger, more fit tennis player so that you can reach your peak performance.

If you follow this plan during the week, you will be at your best when it comes time to play. In fact, you should use the plan's basic concepts before you play (warm up and stretch) *and* after you play (warm down and stretch again). These are the steps that winning tennis players take. They can also help you become a winner and enjoy the sport more.

STEP 1: WARM UP PROPERLY

Warm-up means warming up muscle fibers by increasing your body temperature. This leads to a wide variety of beneficial physiological changes:

- The warmer muscle fibers get, the softer and more fluid they become. They are then able to stretch more easily and to contract more rapidly. The faster a muscle contracts, the stronger it is.

- The higher the temperature of muscle cells, the faster they are able to metabolize the oxygen and fuel they need.

- As muscles warm, the response to nerve impulses quickens, causing faster contraction and, therefore, a quicker response.

- Warming joints lubricates them, allowing them to move more freely with less energy expended. This protects the joints from excessive wear.

- Warm-up gradually increases the heart rate and prevents abnormal heart rhythms. Sudden, strenuous exercise can cause the heart to demand more oxygen than the circulatory system can provide, resulting in a strain on the heart. Studies show that warming up may help prevent the heart attacks that result from abnormal heart rhythms.

How to Warm Up

How do you go about warming up? Before practicing or playing, do light calisthenics, take a brisk walk, jog lightly, ride a stationary bicycle, or do any other easy exercise gradually until you get the heart pumping and thus increase blood flow to your muscles. The goal is to raise the body's temperature by about 2°F, which leads to warm, loose muscles and joints.

You know when your body temperature has gone up because the body has its own natural thermometer: when you break into a sweat, your body temperature has been elevated by about 2°F.

Tennis Warm-up

The United States Tennis Association rule limits the warm-up period to 5 minutes before a match. That's not enough time to practice all of your strokes and to get your body ready for all of the quick movements it needs to make. That's why most professionals find a back court and a practice partner for a pre-warm-up warm-up. The official warm-up then becomes a last-minute drill rather than a comprehensive routine to prepare you for a two-hour match. So if your tennis league follows the letter of the law, try to get in some extra time before the "official" warm-up.

STEP 2: TAKE TIME TO STRETCH

Recreational tennis players tend to stretch first and then begin exercising. However, cold muscles do not stretch well and can pull if overstretched. The best time to stretch is after the body has warmed up. Stretching after warm-up is more likely to lengthen muscles and improve the range of motion of muscles and joints.

Tennis places tremendous demands on different body parts in their extremes of motion—for example, when your arm is fully extended over your head while reaching for a shot. Throughout a match, you are called upon to generate great force from a variety of body positions—changing direction, reaching for a shot, stopping quickly, and serving. A flexible, unrestricted range of motion will help prevent injuries and enhance your performance.

How to Stretch Properly

Bouncing, or ballistic, stretching, can do more damage than not stretching at all. With each bounce, muscle fibers fire and shorten the muscle—the opposite of what you are trying to do. Bouncing actually reduces flexibility.

A static stretch, holding the muscle still for 10 to 20 seconds, is much better. The muscle responds by lengthening slowly.

Each stretch should be gradual and gentle. Try to stretch in a quiet area so that you can concentrate on stretching and not be tempted to rush onto the court. Imagine the muscle gently stretching, the blood pulsing into the muscle, and your body becoming more flexible.

Muscle tightness and injuries can often be traced to hidden areas of inflexibility. This could explain why many tennis players stretch regularly, but see no real gains in flexibility. They may simply be stretching the wrong body parts. When a muscle is tight, it tends to lose sensation, so you may be unaware of the truly tight spots in your body.

Here are some truths that debunk some myths about stretching:

- Being able to touch your toes doesn't necessarily mean that you're flexible. Many traditional stretches have no relationship to actual sports movements. For example, you might have loose hamstrings but tight hips, which can throw off your running stride.

- Lack of flexibility in one area can cause injuries in another. For instance, stiff shoulders that twist, or rotate excessively, can put strain on knees and ankles when you run.

- Flexibility is crucial for good performance. Top athletes aren't necessarily stronger than average, but they do show remarkable range of motion in key areas. Senior tennis player John McEnroe still has great shoulder flexibility, which accounts for his powerful serve.

- Lack of flexibility can be detrimental to performance and general health. If your rib cage is tight, your breathing will be more labored and your posture will be affected, no matter how fit you are. Good flexibility is especially vital in old age. It's because of tightness and inactivity that elderly people's muscles eventually deteriorate.

Warm-up and Warm-down Stretches

The following figures show the proper way to stretch various body parts. Do these stretches for 5 to 10 minutes before and after practicing and playing.

Shoulder Stretch (Arm across Chest)

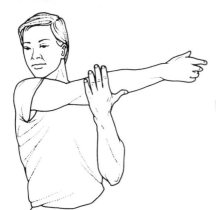

While standing, bring your arm across your chest and pull the elbow gently with the opposite hand. Hold for 20 seconds.

Triceps Stretch

While standing, put your right hand (for right-handers) over your right shoulder with fingers pointing down the back. Place your left hand on your right elbow and gently raise the elbow up, and slide your right hand down your back. Hold for 20 seconds.

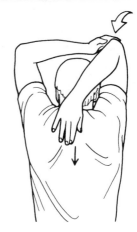

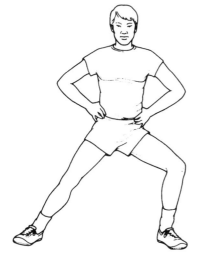

Groin Stretch

Stand with your legs 3 feet apart, hands on hips, and gradually bend your left knee and lean toward your left side. Keep your trunk straight. Hold for 20 seconds. Repeat on the other side.

Hamstring Stretch

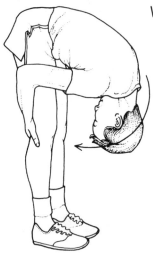

While standing, grab your knees and try to touch your forehead to your knees. Hold for 20 seconds.

Quadriceps Stretch

Stand next to a wall and pull your right foot toward the buttocks with your right hand. Balance yourself against the wall with your left hand. Hold for 20 seconds. Repeat with the other leg.

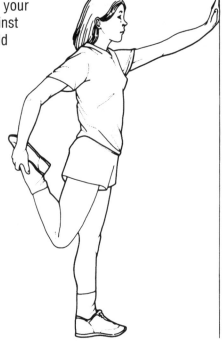

Calf Stretches

Wall Push-up

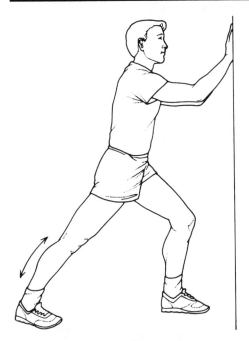

Place one foot as far away from a wall as you can and still keep your rear heel flat on the ground and the other leg a few inches from the wall. Bending your elbows, lean into the wall and support yourself with your hands, but don't let your rear heel come off the ground. Hold the stretch for 20 seconds and push back up. Reverse legs and repeat.

Heel Drop

Stand with your forefeet on a raised surface, as if you were going to do a back dive off a diving board. Let your weight take your heels down below the level of the surface so that the back of your calf is stretched. Hold for 20 seconds and come back up.

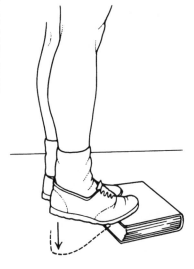

Yoga

Another way to optimize your flexibility and tennis performance is through yoga. Yoga is an excellent regimen to supplement stretching exercises to improve flexibility and help your ability to concentrate and remain calm.

Concentrate on positions that emphasize the legs, shoulders, and lower back. Move through yoga positions slowly and hold each one for several deep breaths. Stop if you feel any pain.

Yoga teaches you to concentrate on your breathing and stay focused, which can come in handy during a long, stressful match. It also keeps joints loose and muscles flexible but strong, which you need when reaching for shots.

Yoga, including newer variations such as fitness yoga and power yoga, involves movements that promote spine agility and balance. Yoga lengthens and strengthens the muscles while reinforcing the connection between the mind and the body.

Yoga classes can be found at special studios or health clubs across the country. Videotapes for beginners to the advanced are also available. One attraction is that you can do yoga in your living room, back porch, or any quiet place. You can also do yoga year-round to maintain your flexibility.

STEP 3: INCLUDE AGILITY AND SPEED TRAINING

Your ability to move around the court quickly and smoothly to position yourself for a shot depends on agility and speed. Agility is crucial to good court movement. It allows you to be in the correct position and provides a solid platform from which to hit the ball. Speed is important to get to the ball. The faster you can get to the ball, the more time you have to prepare for the shot.

Tennis requires a variety of movement and footwork. Lateral movement is important as well as changing from a shuffle step to a sprint step. You also have to lunge for a shot, followed by a rapid return to the ready position.

The following self-tests will help you get a baseline level of your speed and agility. Do these tests twice a week and you will quickly see an improvement in your quickness.

20-Yard Dash

This test measures the time it takes to go 20 yards from a standing position. Your score is in seconds. It measures both velocity and acceleration.

Velocity is how fast you go at any one time. Acceleration is your ability to get going up to that speed.

Acceleration is an important part of tennis because many times you take the shot from nearly a stopped position.

To improve velocity and acceleration, use line sprints from one line to another on the court. Work on getting up to speed as fast as possible and then maintain your speed.

Spider Test

The spider test measures the time it takes to pick up five tennis balls that are spread across the court and return them individually to a specified zone such as the baseline. It records your agility and speed. Your score is in seconds.

In this test, you are allowed to face in any direction and move in whatever direction possible. The spider test includes stopping, starting, and changing direction. It also includes vertical motion (bending your knees to pick up and put down balls).

Use the spider test to work on stopping, starting, and bending your knees.

Sideways Shuffle

The sideways shuffle measures the time it takes to shuffle your feet to each of the doubles sidelines and back to the center service line. Your score is in seconds.

This test measures your ability to move laterally. Fast lateral movements occur very frequently during a tennis match. Many times you are forced to stop moving laterally in one step to prepare for the next stroke. This test uses lateral motion to both sides.

Notice whether a sideways shuffle is harder or slower in one direction than the other, and work harder and more frequently in the direction of your more difficult side.

STEP 4: ADD IN CONDITIONING
AND STRENGTH TRAINING

Once you have warmed up and stretched, you can begin your tennis game. You will be prepared because you have warmed up and stretched. But you will be even better prepared to play if you have included agility and speed work. Now it's time to add in conditioning and strength training as well.

Conditioning

Tennis is aces when it comes to providing a total aerobic workout. To work on conditioning, pros will do upper-body strength training at the gym, foot drills in the sand, sprints on the volleyball court, and then run 2 miles daily. Good physical conditioning allows you to have solid footwork so you can get to the ball on balance and have a sound foundation for hitting ground strokes.

As with any exercise, you will burn calories when you play tennis. How many calories you burn depends on your gender, your fitness, and the intensity, frequency, and type of game you play. For instance, a woman will burn approximately 400 calories playing one hour of singles, but only half that amount playing doubles. A man will burn approximately 600 calories playing singles and only 400 calories playing doubles.

Your physical fitness plays a role, too. If you are in good physical condition it will be easier to play the game. You'll be less prone to injuries and you'll have more endurance. But if you are in poor physical condition, you will gain extra aerobic benefits from tennis. You'll work harder to get to the ball (although you'll also get winded faster). The more intensely you play, the more calories you will burn for each hour of tennis. The more frequently you play, the more total calories you will burn.

If you are a regular tournament player, you will burn more calories than if you are a weekend warrior. But a weekend warrior will burn more calories playing intensely than a social player.

Tennis can improve the way a person handles a stressful situation. Tennis's soothing effects can be attributed to the endorphins and catecholamines, the body's natural stress-reducers, that are released during play. Moreover, the interval-like training associated with tennis helps the body respond to stress.

Aerobic Endurance

Aerobic energy is used during prolonged, steady-paced activities, mainly using the large muscle groups. When you are aerobically fit, you can recover faster between points and perform longer before getting tired.

To build aerobic endurance, you need to work your heart at 70 to 85 percent of maximum for 20 to 30 minutes at a time. Begin with high volume and low intensity, such as jogging, then gradually progress to increased intensity and lower volume, such as interval training. Interval training consists of going hard for a short burst in the middle of a lengthy aerobic activity. For example, you might sprint during a jogging session.

The following program shows you how to do interval training while running. I suggest that you start by sprinting 50 yards for every mile you jog. Gradually increase the sprint distance by 100 yards per mile. Then increase the number of sprints—go 100 yards for every half mile. Once you feel comfortable at that level, sprint 200 yards for every half mile.

Now you are ready to take the final step. Jog one mile and then run a 200-yard sprint. Jog for 200 yards, or about 30 seconds, and then sprint another 200 yards. Continue jogging and sprinting 200 yards eight times to complete a mile. Then continue jogging to finish your workout.

This is the type of interval training that the New York Giants players do. We have them sprint back and forth across the width of the field, resting 30 seconds between sprints. They do four sprints, each one faster than the previous one, to build up their speed.

Elite athletes often spend a full aerobic workout doing only speed work. The recreational athlete can simply put interval training in the middle of an aerobic workout and gradually increase the distance and speed. I suggest that you alternate doing long, slow aerobic workouts with interval training aerobic workouts to build both cardiovascular conditioning and speed.

Keep training year-round, if possible, to avoid becoming deconditioned. The average tennis player will lose 50 percent of aerobic endurance within three weeks of inactivity. In the off-season, jog 2 to 3 miles, three times a week. In the preseason, run a total of ten 220-yard dashes, resting for 45 seconds in between each one, three to four times a week. During the season, do sprint and agility drills one to three times a week.

Strength Training

Few of us have a serve that is explosive, powerful, and deadly accurate. Tennis players generally aren't known for their muscles. Yet players who ignore strength training put themselves at a competitive disadvantage, since well-toned muscles can help them hit the ball harder and charge the net faster. Muscle strengthening also reduces the risk of injury from overuse, which is as much of a problem for occasional players as for the pros.

The best way to improve your tennis game is not simply to play more tennis. You need a total-body strength-training program to help you hit the ball harder, move faster, and beat the players who are now beating you. In tennis, muscle strength has to be accompanied by muscle stamina. That is built by using light weights and doing many repetitions. Top players now travel with strength-training coaches to enhance their games.

Like all sports, tennis emphasizes a limited number of muscle groups. Even in your serving arm, certain muscles tend to be neglected. This can result in injury to the overworked muscles. Strength training, by compensating for these muscle imbalances, may prevent tendinitis or other damage. Strengthening the shoulder helps prevent rotator cuff injuries. And if tennis players would strengthen their forearm and wrist muscles, they wouldn't get tennis elbow.

Power

Power is the underlying essence of tennis. Surprisingly, most tennis players don't train themselves to become more powerful. Power improves quickness and enables you to have a strong serve and return. Combined with skill work and conditioning, power training can make your game more competitive.

Tennis requires you to make explosive movements. Greater power allows you to respond quicker and produce forceful movements with less effort. Players with explosive first steps get into position quickly, set up well, and hit effective shots. In addition, an explosive first step will give you the speed necessary to get to balls hit further away.

Generating Power

To develop explosive power, you must follow a sequence of movements common to all sports. Start the sequence by using your feet against the tennis court to move energy from muscles in the legs to the trunk and finally to the arms. Rotate your body so that all of the large muscle groups stretch, then rapidly unwind. The arms and racquet should be left behind. You can generate tremendous velocity when you let the arms and racquet move in a coordinated fashion with the legs and trunk.

The hips must also rotate toward your target to get more power. Early hip rotation is one way to add power, but you must not open up the hips too soon. This causes your weight to shift forward before your arm has time to catch up and hit the ball.

Recreational tennis players may be able to generate lower-body power, but often have trouble transmitting that power to the racquet.

The shoulder muscles may be the weak link. When your larger lower-body muscles are firing toward the target, they have to drag the arms along. The best tennis swing unwinds so that the racquet accelerates just as the shoulders come in line with the ball.

Stronger shoulders are important, but not as important as improving your swing mechanics. The best tennis players have great mechanics in delivering the racquet head to the ball. You don't have to be big to be powerful. Good swing mechanics will do more to add a little zip to your shots.

Both lower- and upper-body power are necessary in tennis. To increase lower-body power, do sprints, particularly uphill. Also, do jumping, or plyometric, exercises. For the upper body, do medicine ball tosses, working with a partner, as top players Lindsay Davenport and Patrick Rafter do.

Plyometric Exercises

Hop over Bench and Dash

Use a bench or step that is low enough for you to jump over, but high enough to be a challenge, generally up to 30 inches. Face the bench with your feet shoulder width apart, then hop over the bench. As soon as you land, dash to the right for a few steps as if you were reaching for an impossible shot way off to the side of the court. Return to the bench, hop over, and run to the left a few steps. Repeat until your muscles are fatigued.

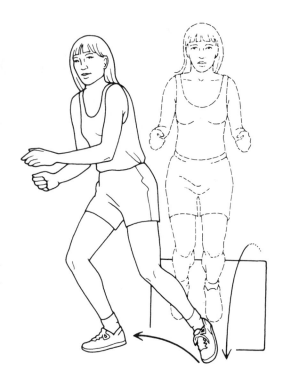

Lateral Cone Hop

Place two plastic cones, about 2 feet tall, about 6 feet apart. Jump sideways over one cone and then the other, landing on both feet. After the last cone, change direction by pushing off on the outside foot. Repeat until your muscles are fatigued.

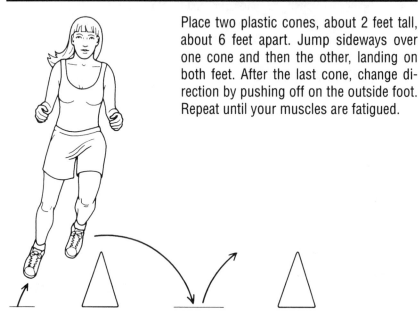

Medicine Ball Exercises

Medicine Ball Catch and Toss

Sit on a bench across from a partner, who also is sitting. Grab a medicine ball with two hands and bring it over your head. Bend your elbows until they point at the ceiling and toss the ball to your partner, who catches the ball, lowers it behind the head, and tosses it back to you as quickly as possible. Don't push from your fingers. Use your arms, chest, and shoulder muscles as if you were serving or returning a lob. Your upper body should bend forward a little as you toss the ball. Build up to three sets of 8 to 10 repetitions.

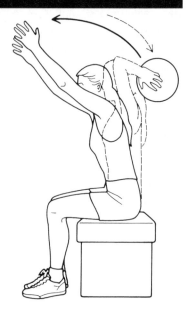

Strength and Endurance

Strength is the amount of weight you can lift or handle at any one time. Muscular endurance is the number of times your muscles can lift a weight or how long your muscles can hold an amount of weight. By increasing strength, you can increase the amount of force with which you hit the ball. By increasing endurance, you will be able to perform movements as well at the end of a match as you did at the beginning.

Training with weights is the quickest, most efficient way to develop both strength and endurance. Great strength is a prerequisite for power. To move explosively, you need a certain amount of pure strength that is not specific to tennis. As you gain strength, you will find that you can hit the ball harder and more accurately, plus you won't get tired as quickly.

Strength training also helps to prevent injury. The shocks and stresses tennis places on the joints can be reduced by strengthening the supporting muscles, ligaments, and tendons.

A Strength-Training Program

The following strength-training program gives you exercises for the chest, shoulders, back, legs, calves, thighs, abdominals, biceps, and triceps. Try to work different muscles on different days, and intersperse light and heavy repetitions. For example, follow a light Day 1 program Monday and a light Day 2 program Tuesday. Rest on Wednesday. Then on Thursday and Friday alternate heavy programs. Remember to warm up and stretch before even light repetitions, and to warm down and stretch at the end of each workout.

Start off using enough weight so that you can comfortably do 12 repetitions of an exercise on a light day. For example, if you can bench-press 80 pounds 20 times, then you need to move up to a slightly heavier weight, say 90 pounds. Once you have found the right weight to accomplish 12 repetitions of each exercise, move on to a heavy workout and use 20 percent more weight. To compensate for the greater weight, do fewer repetitions.

Once you can very easily do 12 repetitions of an exercise on a light day, increase the amount of weight by 5 percent for both light and heavy workouts. You must be able to do 12 repetitions at the greater weight for a light workout, or else you should drop back down to the previous weight. If you follow this program regularly, each month you should be able to add about 5 percent more weight.

Strength-Training Program

Exercise	Number of Sets	Number of Repetitions	
		Light Day	Heavy Day
Day 1			
Chest			
Bench Press	3–4	12	6–8
Flat Fly	3	12	8–10
Shoulders			
Upright Row	3	12	6–8
Lateral Raise	3	12	8–10
Triceps			
Triceps Extension	3–4	12	8–10
Kickback	3	12	8–10
Abdominals			
Decline Sit-up	2–3	20	15
Standing Crunch	2–3	20	15
Calves			
Standing Raise	3	15–20	15–20
Day 2			
Legs			
Leg Press	4	12	6–8
Leg Extension	3	15	10
Leg Curl	3	15	10
Thigh Burner	3	12–15	10–15
Back			
Wide-Grip Rear Chin-up	3	12	8–10
Bent-over Rowing	3	12	8–10
Biceps			
Seated Curl	3	12	8–10
Barbell Curl	3	12	8–10
Abdominals, Calves			
Same as Day 1			

You will notice from the Strength-Training Program chart that exercises for both the abdominals and calves are included in each workout day. These muscles are difficult to build up and need to be exercised each day you work out. On a light day, you can do fewer abdominal exercises, but you need to work your calves virtually to exhaustion to strengthen them.

In the off-season, do three to four sets of each exercise, 5 to 12 repetitions, at moderate intensity, at least once a week. In the preseason, increase to a higher intensity and do three sets, at least twice a week. During the season, do two sets once or twice a week to maintain your muscular strength. Muscular endurance is a combination of muscular strength and aerobic endurance. Work on those two and you will improve your muscular endurance as well.

One warning: Don't lift weights and then go out and play tennis. You temporarily lose some fine motor control when you lift weights, and you also tire out muscles. Lift on the days you don't play, or lift after you have played.

Strength-Training Exercises

Chest

Bench Press

Lie on your back on a bench with feet flat on the floor while holding a barbell at the top of your chest. Press the weight straight up, pause, and then return it back down. Barely touch your chest and start the next repetition.

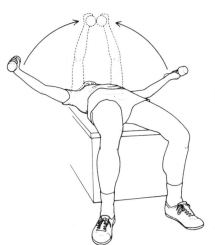

Flat Fly

Lie on your back on a bench with feet flat on the floor while holding dumbbells out to the sides, arms bent slightly. Push the dumbbells overhead in a semicircular motion until they touch. Pause and then return to the starting position.

Shoulders

Upright Row

Grasp a barbell with palms down in front of you about shoulder width apart. Bring the bar up beneath your chin, extending your elbows out to the sides. Pause and then return to the starting position.

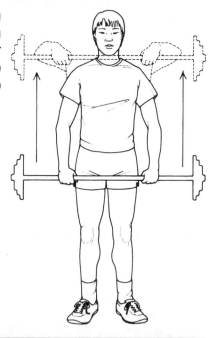

Lateral Raise

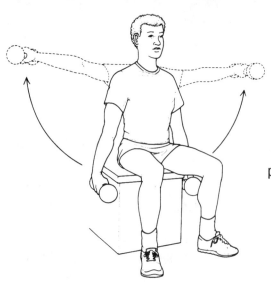

Sit on a bench with a dumbbell in each hand. With palms facing down, keep both arms straight and slowly raise them to shoulder level. Pause and then slowly lower your arms to the starting position.

Triceps

Triceps Extension

Stand holding a barbell overhead, palms facing up and elbows bent. Lower the bar behind you, keeping your upper arms stationary. Pause at the bottom and then bring the bar back up to the starting position.

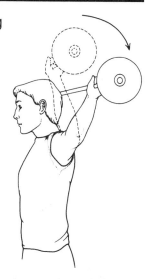

Kickback

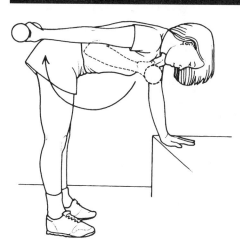

While standing, bend at the waist and support yourself with one hand on a bench. Grasp a dumbbell with the other hand and hold it with your lower arm parallel to the floor. Keeping your upper arm stationary, bring the weight straight back. Pause and return to the starting position.

Abdominals

Decline Sit-up

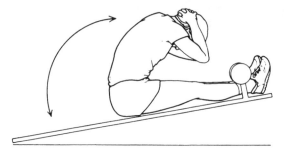

Lie on your back on an inclined board with your feet above your head and hooked under the pads. With hands behind your head and chin touching your chest, sit up until your elbows touch lightly. Lower yourself back down to the starting position.

Standing Crunch

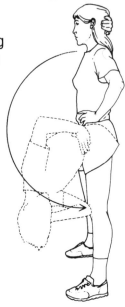

Stand with your right hand behind your head. Bring your right elbow down to meet your left knee while crunching your abdominal muscles. Pause and return to the starting position. Do the appropriate number of repetitions and then repeat with the opposite hand and knee.

Calves

Standing Raise

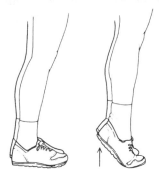

Place a barbell on top of your shoulders or position your shoulders under the bars of an upright calf machine. With only the balls of your feet on the floor or on the platform, raise up onto your toes, pause, and then return to the starting position.

Legs

Leg Press

Sit on an inclined or regular leg press machine and press the weight until your legs are almost (but not quite) straight. Pause and then slowly lower the weight to the starting position.

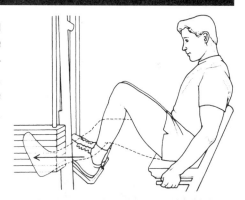

Leg Extension

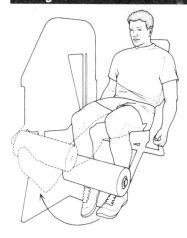

Sit on a bench or leg extension machine with your legs at a 90° angle and your feet flexed (soles parallel to the floor). Hold the bottom of the bench for support and rapidly lift the weight with one leg to full extension (toes pointing up). Pause and then bring your leg back down. Do the appropriate number of repetitions, and then repeat with the other leg.

Leg Curl

Lie face down on a bench with your head over the edge. Hold the bottom of the bench for support. Begin with your right leg straight and left leg bent at the knee, foot flexed. Lift the weight up as high as possible with

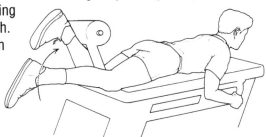

your left thigh while keeping your right leg on the bench. Pause at the top and then lower your leg. Do the appropriate number of repetitions, and then repeat with the other leg.

Thigh Burner

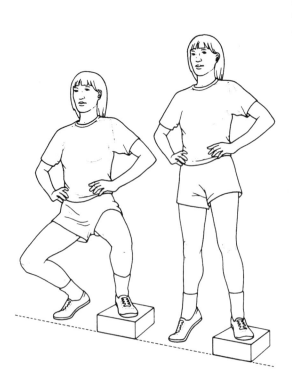

Stand on a step or a thick telephone book with your left foot fully on the step in a 10 o'clock position and your right foot in a 2 o'clock position with the heel off the floor. Place your hands on your hips and slowly lower yourself down, keeping the right heel off the floor, until your left thigh is parallel to the floor. Almost all of your weight should be on your right thigh. Then push back up to the starting position. Do the appropriate number of repetitions, and then repeat with the other leg.

Back

Wide-Grip Rear Chin-up

Grasp a bar above your head with a grip wider than shoulder width, palms out. Bend your legs at the knees and cross your feet, then pull yourself up until the bar touches the back of your neck. Pause and then lower yourself back down.

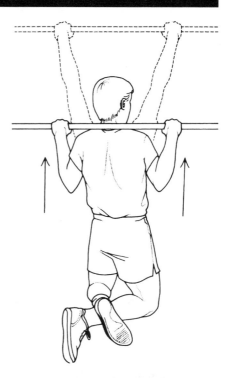

Bent-over Rowing

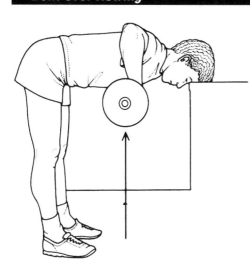

Place a barbell on the floor in front of a bench at waist level. Place your forehead on the bench for support, reach down, and grasp the barbell with both hands in a wide grip. Bring the barbell up until it touches your chest. Pause and then return it back down.

Biceps

Seated Curl

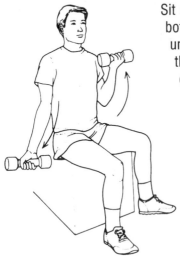

Sit at the end of a bench with dumbbells in both hands, palms up. Curl one dumbbell up until your forearm touches your biceps and then lower it. As you lower the dumbbell, curl the other one up. The two dumbbells should reach the starting and top positions simultaneously.

Barbell Curl

Stand and hold a barbell at arms' length with your hands shoulder width apart, palms out. Curl the bar up until it is under your chin. Pause and return to the starting position.

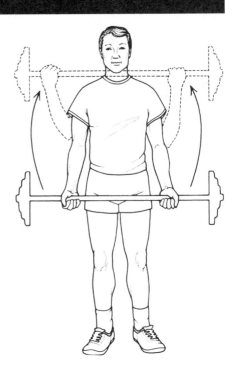

STEP 5: WARM DOWN GRADUALLY

I use the term "warm down" instead of "cool down" to indicate that this step is the reverse of the warm-up. The body naturally cools down by itself at the end of activity. The warm-down is a 5 to 10 minute period of continued, mild activity after strenuous exercise.

A gradual warm-down allows your heart to slow down and adjust its blood flow without any pooling of blood in the muscles. Say you're out jogging and have just finished a run of several miles, and you stop suddenly. While you were running, the blood vessels to your muscles dilated to increase the blood supply of oxygen and fuel to the muscles. At the same time, your heart rate rose rapidly as the heart pumped more blood to the muscles. So the blood vessels to your legs are now wide open, and your heart is pumping blood down to your legs.

The body depends on a massaging action of contracting and relaxing muscles on the veins to return blood from the legs back up to the heart. When you suddenly stop your heart rate remains high for a short while, and blood keeps pumping down to your legs. Without the massaging action of your leg muscles, there will be very little return flow to the heart, and large amounts of blood will pool in your legs. This may not leave enough blood to supply your brain or hardworking heart, and this can lead to fainting or even a heart attack, particularly if you're an older player.

But if you keep moving after running, or playing a match, the massaging action will pump blood back to the heart until your heart rate has returned to normal and your body's blood vessels have returned to normal size. Simply walking for 5 to 10 minutes is usually enough.

Warm-down also enhances the removal of lactic acid from muscles, which reduces muscle soreness. Lactic acid builds up in muscles as a by-product of anaerobic metabolism after the body's primary energy source (glycogen) has been exhausted. Keeping the blood flowing through muscles during warm-down washes lactic acid out of the muscles.

"Pumping Up"

During a strength-training workout, circulation to straining muscles increases markedly, causing the muscles to swell. This is the "pump" that weight lifters delight in, a sign that the muscles are working hard.

Strength training is basically an anaerobic exercise. If a large amount of blood pools in muscles, as it does during the pump, then the lactic acid remains in the muscles.

The gradually decreasing exercise of the warm-down period massages out the pooled blood as the muscles contract. The blood moves back to the heart and takes the lactic acid with it. So if you are doing an upper-body workout, use light dumbbells to keep your muscles moving as you warm down. If you are doing a lower-body workout, simply walk around to keep the blood flowing in the muscles. If you are working the whole body, use dumbbells as you walk around.

STEP 6: STRETCH AGAIN

Stretching your muscles after the warm-down helps restore full range of motion and flexibility and reduces the likelihood of tearing a muscle during your next workout or tennis match. Restretching muscles after exercise can also prevent soreness and stiffness. Exercised muscles tend to shorten. If left that way, they will be stiff and sore the following day. Still-warm muscles can be restretched easily during warm-down to alleviate any annoying stiffness.

So after you have warmed down, or played a match, go through the same stretching program you used after warming up. You will find that those 10 to 20 minutes of stretching after warm-up and warm-down will go a long way toward preventing injuries, muscle soreness, and stiffness. This may be the most important time you spend during your entire workout.

REHABILITATION OF TENNIS INJURIES

The rehabilitation of tennis injuries should ensure the full restoration of function of both the injured area as well as each link in the swing. A gradual return to activity and avoiding any previous training errors are important to prevent any reinjuries. Avoiding excessive practice, along with improved biomechanics, should reduce your incidence of tennis injuries.

The following rehabilitation program should get you back on the courts after a tennis injury. A good warm-up is an essential part of any sports activity, including tennis. So warm up for 10 minutes before going through your rehabilitation routine.

Don't progress or continue the program if you feel any joint pain. Always stretch the shoulder, elbow, and wrist of the dominant arm (right for right-handers) before and after the program. Ice these joints afterward for about 20 minutes if you feel pain in them. Do the program every other day, giving your body a day of rest between sessions. Don't progress to the next phase if you feel pain or excessive fatigue during your last outing.

Preliminary Stage

Using a foam ball, have a partner standing at the net feed you 20 to 25 forehand and backhand strokes.

First Stage

Using a regular tennis ball, have a partner feed you 20 forehands from the net, followed by 20 backhands. The tossed balls should be looping and waist-high.

Rest for 5 minutes.

Hit 20 forehands and 20 backhands again.

Second Stage

Repeat the first stage, then rally from the baseline, hitting 50 controlled ground strokes. Mix in forehands and backhands.

Rest for 5 minutes.

Hit 50 more controlled ground strokes.

Third Stage

Hit ground strokes from the baseline for 5 minutes.

Rest for 5 minutes.

Hit 10 forehand volleys and 10 backhand volleys, making sure to hit the ball in front of your body.

Rally for 15 minutes from the baseline.

Hit 10 more forehand volleys and 10 backhand volleys.

Pre-Serve Stage

Stretch your shoulder, elbow, and wrist while holding a racquet.

Perform your serving motion 10 to 15 times without hitting a ball.

Using a foam ball, hit 10 to 15 serves. Concentrate on the form of your racquet arm and contact point.

Fourth Stage

Hit 20 minutes of ground strokes, mixing in volleys. Hit twice as many ground strokes as volleys.

Hit 10 serves.
Rest for 5 minutes.
Hit 10 to 15 more serves.
Hit ground strokes for 5 to 10 minutes.

Fifth Stage

Hit 20 minutes of ground strokes, mixing in volleys. Hit twice as many ground strokes as volleys.

Hit 10 serves.
Hit 5 to 10 easy, short overhead smashes.
Hit ground strokes for 5 to 10 minutes.

2

Eat to Compete

While I was attending a medical meeting in Monaco, I stopped by the Monaco Tennis Club, made famous by Bjorn Borg, to watch a friendly match between two colleagues on center court. Near the end of the first set, I noticed that one player was running out of gas on this hot summer day. So I went inside the clubhouse and ordered an orange juice, watered it down a bit, then added a little salt and a dollop of honey. At the next service break, I had the nearly exhausted player take the drink. He lost that set, but felt replenished and took the next two sets. He went home with a new respect for proper fluid intake, as well as *"le Clay de Borg"* on his tennis shoes.

Eating right is imperative for championship athletes, but anyone can gain an edge by knowing the best foods to eat and when to eat them.

What's the best thing for tennis players to eat? Most dietary advice buzzed around the locker room is exaggerated, inaccurate, or downright harmful. This chapter dispels some of those myths and offers solid advice on which to build a better body for tennis:

- Eat a winning diet combination.
- What to eat in the off-season.
- What to eat before, during, and after playing.
- What to drink before, during, and after playing.

THE WINNING DIET COMBINATION

To perform your best on the tennis court, you should eat a balanced diet of low-fat, moderate-protein, high-carbohydrate foods and beverages; snack on high-carbohydrate, low-fat foods; and drink plenty of fluids. Good nutrition can help you reach your athletic potential.

Within a balanced diet, choose these lower-fat items whenever possible:

- Have a slice of whole wheat bread, an English muffin, a bagel, or a nongranola cereal without nuts or seeds, such as Cheerios, Wheaties, or cornflakes.

- Eat fresh, whole fruits, which are better for weight loss because they contain more fiber than juices. Drink 100 percent fruit juice rather than juice drinks.

- Develop a taste for low-fat dairy products such as skim or 1 percent milk.

- Choose brightly colored vegetables and fresh or frozen vegetables without added fat because they have more vitamins and are more nutritious.

- Eat fish, seafood, and poultry more often than beef and other red meats. Eat lean cuts of well-trimmed meat with little marbling. Have poultry without the skin and nonbreaded and nonfried whenever possible.

- Use reduced-fat margarine, mayonnaise, and salad dressing. Use canola or olive oil and salad dressing without cream or cheese. Take in fat primarily in the form of fish, canola oil, or olive oil.

Emphasize Carbohydrates

A diet high in carbohydrates, moderate in proteins, and low in fats can also help keep your energy level up during a weight loss program. Carbohydrates also have a fair amount of fiber, so they fill you up with fewer calories. A lot of fatty foods contain fat and fat-soluble vitamins, but nothing else. Many foods high in carbohydrates have small amounts of protein and a number of vitamins and minerals. Sources of carbohydrates include breads, cereals, grains, and other starches such as potatoes, corn, milk, beans, peas, lentils, fruits and fruit juices, and vegetables.

Without a doubt, carbohydrates are the best foods for tennis players to sustain training and competition, promote rapid recovery, and prevent staleness and fatigue.

Remember Protein

Although protein can not be metabolized for energy, it contains amino acids, the building blocks for body tissue.

In tennis, as in any active sport, there is a breakdown of body tissue. The continued use of muscle fibers breaks them down, and the body needs protein to repair them.

While children need a relatively high level of protein in their diets because they are still growing, adults need only enough protein to maintain tissue repair.

OFF-SEASON NUTRITION

Weight control is very important to better tennis. Carrying around excess weight cuts down on your speed and stamina. Tennis is also a game of quickness as well as speed. Being overweight makes it harder to get your body started toward the ball. Sudden changes in direction are much more difficult with a larger body mass.

The off-season is a good time to control weight. To do that, you need to consume fewer calories and eat a low-fat diet. Fat (with 9 calories per gram) has more than twice as many calories as carbohydrates and proteins (4 calories per gram). Weight loss depends on a simple equation: calories in should be less than calories out. By reducing the calorie intake of your diet and increasing your calorie expenditure with exercise, you will lose weight.

If you play year-round, you will basically have to watch your weight all of the time.

WHAT TO EAT BEFORE, DURING, AND AFTER PLAYING

Before Hitting a Ball

Tennis demands a huge amount of energy. Your body utilizes its carbohydrate stores for this energy. Once the carbohydrates are exhausted, your body switches to burning fat. This is much less efficient in producing energy. So the more carbohydrates you have stored in your body, the longer you can play before your body shifts to the less effective energy mode.

Ideally, you should eat a high-carbohydrate meal about 3 to 4 hours before playing. Before a big match, because of added anxiety, allow more time than normal. Being nervous slows down digestion, and you may become more aware of stomach upset. This may be tolerable during a practice session or your regular game, but it could affect your performance in a tournament.

Before going out onto the court, eat a high-carbohydrate meal. I prefer a bowl of high-fiber cereal, fruit, and low-fat milk before an early morning match. Early morning tennis players tend to skip breakfast because they don't want to play on a full stomach. While a full stomach may interfere with performance, if you have not eaten since the evening before, all ready sources of energy from carbohydrates will have already been depleted, and your performance will suffer even more. Basically, you need to leave enough time so that food empties from your stomach, yet eat close enough to your playing time to prevent hunger and exhaustion later on. At the least, eat a piece of fruit and either a high-energy bar or drink.

Avoid high-fat foods before playing. Foods high in fat slow the emptying time of the stomach by several hours. The body responds to exercising muscles by sending them an increased supply of blood that contains nutrients. However, the intestinal tract gets first priority after you have eaten. So a full stomach gets the increased blood supply to aid digestion, not the muscles.

During the Match

A high-energy bar is a good choice, and much better than a candy bar. High-energy bars are derivatives of granola bars, with much of the fat removed and more carbohydrates added in. Nutritionally, they are far superior to candy bars.

Candy bars taste good, but they have several drawbacks. Their high-fat content contributes to delayed emptying of the stomach. This not only reduces the amount of energy available to working muscles, but delays needed energy from reaching the muscles. Candy bars also rely on sugar for energy rather than complex carbohydrates. A sudden increase in circulating blood sugar causes the body to respond by secreting a large amount of insulin. This overproduction of insulin burns up stored carbohydrates, leaving you with lower stores than if you did nothing. An energy bar does not trigger the surge in insulin.

At every changeover, take a few sips of a sports drink with a high carbohydrate content, which will help replenish carbohydrate stores.

In the Clubhouse

After playing, the most important thing for a tennis player to do is to replenish fluids. Drink plain old water or a sports drink. Within 2 hours of exercise, and preferably within 15 minutes, have a high-carbohydrate drink as well. Taking in quick carbohydrates within that time frame seems to accelerate the replacement of muscle glycogen reserves.

When you rehydrate, limit caffeinated drinks such as coffee, cola, and iced tea. This can be hard to do because you're tired, and a quick shot of caffeine makes you feel better. But if you drink too much caffeine, you will urinate more and lose fluids. The same goes for alcohol, which goes through your body as if it were a leaky tub. Limit yourself to two drinks or less of caffeine or alcohol a day because both promote water loss.

Within a few hours after playing, eat a good, balanced meal. The food should include enough protein to allow tissues to repair themselves after exercising. The average American eats seven times as much protein as is necessary, so most tennis players do not need to eat anything extra or insist on a steak. The amount of calories replaced depends on the amount of energy expended, which is typically based on whether you played singles or doubles. A tennis player may burn between 1,000 calories (doubles) to 2,000 calories (singles).

There is no special diet for tennis players. Most of the replacement calories after playing should come from complex carbohydrates, such as potatoes, bread, green vegetables, and fruit. Again, try to avoid fats and sweets.

WHAT TO DRINK BEFORE, DURING AND AFTER PLAYING

A tennis player's concerns about fluid intake and hydration depend on heat and humidity. An increase in either temperature or humidity can cause body heat problems. Humidity is more important than temperature. However, a day with high temperature and low humidity may be deceiving. Sweat evaporates so rapidly that you may not be aware of fluid loss. With high humidity, sweat evaporates more slowly, so at least most tennis players are more aware of sweating.

In high temperature and high humidity, tennis players need to begin drinking approximately one hour before playing—about 8 ounces of liquid every 20 minutes. During your warm-up, drink cold water. Cold water empties from the stomach faster than warm water. If you have stomach cramps, it's probably from taking too much water at once. If you experience cramps, try warm water or fluids with salt or sugar in them.

Drink water at every changeover, if possible. Have a water bottle with you at courtside. Don't wait until thirst sets in. You will never catch up. Continue to take in liquids after coming off the court.

As the body depletes its supply of fluid, muscles lose their flexibility and strength. The end result of fluid deprivation can be heat exhaustion and heatstroke. If you are going to play daily in a hot, humid climate, such as on a tennis vacation, weigh yourself daily. If your weight stays constant, you are replacing lost liquids adequately.

It takes about 7 to 10 days to acclimate to heat. After that, the body learns to conserve fluids. Unfortunately, most tennis vacations last just about that long, so be aware of losing weight rapidly. A tennis player who loses more than three pounds of body weight over a few days may be becoming dehydrated and runs the risk of having difficulty with muscle cramps and heat illness (see chapter 4). Drinking more than the normal amount of water can get the weight back up.

Electrolyte Replacement

A loss of electrolytes (salt and potassium) leads to muscle cramping and fatigue. You need some salt to compensate for sweat losses, but there is no place for salt pills in tennis, or any sport for that matter. A large amount of salt in the intestines causes the body to extract large amounts of water from the body tissues to dilute it, causing further dehydration in the muscles.

In hot weather, simply eat more salty foods, like pickles and relish. Check with your doctor if you are on a salt-restricted diet. Also, eat more high potassium foods, such as bananas, tomatoes, melons, and skim milk. These high-potassium foods are also good because they are great sources of carbohydrates and proteins, contain no fat, and provide lots of vitamins and minerals.

Sports drinks contain all of the electrolytes, plus liquid and glucose, necessary for energy replacement.

GAIN MUSCLE, LOSE EXCESS FAT

Gaining muscle and losing fat makes you stronger. Therefore, all tennis players should strive to gain muscle and lose fat. To do so, you need to increase your calorie intake through a combination of low-fat, high-protein and low-fat, high-carbohydrate foods and beverages.

Losing Weight

The goals of any weight loss program should be to lose excess body fat while maintaining muscle and keeping up fluid intake. Any program that significantly depletes muscle mass or fluids isn't healthy, and will not be effective for long-term weight control.

Tennis players may get excited when they lose 2 pounds after a long day on the courts. But this sudden weight loss usually is due to loss of fluids, which you will need to replenish. Losing excess fluid is counterproductive because it lowers the body's volume of blood. The blood circulates oxygen to working muscles and takes waste products away. With a lower blood volume, you can't do that as efficiently. In addition, your heart has to work harder to keep the blood circulating. A low blood volume also reduces your sweat volume so that your body doesn't cool off as quickly.

A weight loss of 1 to 2 pounds of fat per week through combined diet and exercise is feasible. Any more than that and you are probably losing muscle and fluid, not body fat.

The best way to lose body fat is to decrease your intake of food fats *and* increase aerobic exercise. This dynamic duo is not only the best program for training, performance, and weight control, but for overall general health as well.

A Weight Loss Diet

Where do fats appear in our food? We get fats from meat, fish, poultry, cooking fat and oil, butter and margarine, mayonnaise and salad dressing, nut and nut butter, whole milk, cream, most cheeses, ice cream, nondairy creamers, pastries, cake, donuts, pies, cookies, chips, and other greasy snacks. A simple way of testing if a food is fatty is to put it on a paper napkin. If it leaves a grease spot, you know it's full of fat.

To lose weight, you need to cut down on the portions of high-fat foods you eat. When you do eat fat, try to have it in nutritious foods.

One way to lose weight is to replace some fats with carbohydrates. A registered dietitian can help point out high-fat foods and offer lower fat alternatives. For example, switch from eating donuts (high fat) to bagels (low fat), or from ice cream (high fat) to frozen yogurt (low fat).

Plugging in a suitable, tasty alternative makes a long-term behavior change doable. Most people hate sitting down to wimpy food portions. By eating lower-fat foods, you can still have fairly large portions and eat when you're hungry.

Part Two

Common Risks and Basic Safeguards

First Aid: What to Do until the Doctor Comes

Medical Risks

Health Gadgets

First Aid: What to Do until the Doctor Comes

The first person to treat an injured professional athlete is usually the team physician or trainer. Unfortunately, most amateur athletes are treated by someone who has no training or little, if any, experience in administering first aid to sports injuries.

The two basic principles of immediate first aid are to protect the athlete from further injury and to get the athlete back in action as soon and safely as possible. To be sure this happens, every recreational athlete needs to follow these basic principles:

- Take your time.
- Use the RICE formula to reduce swelling.
- Note how the injury happened.
- Use the right painkillers.
- Use first aid for common muscle injuries.

TAKE YOUR TIME

If you become injured, take your time. Don't allow yourself to be rushed off the court. You may feel as if you have to get to the sideline as quickly as possible. Well-meaning but inexperienced friends or officials may pressure you to get on with the game.

Don't be pressured into moving before you are convinced that it's safe. Also, take care about walking off the court. Many recreational athletes believe that once an athlete is on her feet, she will be okay. But I have seen athletes walk off the court only to collapse when they get to the sideline. Lie still until you are absolutely sure it's safe to move. If you are not sure, wait for a stretcher.

USE THE RICE FORMULA TO REDUCE SWELLING

The most basic treatment principle is summed up by the acronym RICE, which stands for *r*est, *i*ce, *c*ompression and *e*levation. These four components of treatment, used in combination, reduce swelling, which occurs when blood and fluids leak into the injured body part, often a joint.

Swelling is the most important factor in delaying your return to activity long after the pain is gone. A swollen joint has severely limited function. If you can keep the swelling down to a minimum at the time of injury, then you will have much less pain and aggravation to deal with as you heal. Anything that can prevent swelling will save you days of recovery later on.

Resting the injury cuts down the circulation to the area. The less circulation, the less leaking from broken blood vessels. Also, when small blood vessels are torn, any motion in the area prevents them from sealing off, so they keep bleeding.

Ice constricts blood vessels when first applied. The blood vessels shrink down and limit bleeding into the affected area, which reduces swelling.

Compressing the swollen area with an elastic bandage limits the area available for fluid to leak into. Compression causes a higher pressure outside of the torn blood vessels than inside, which makes it difficult for fluid to flow out.

Elevating the damaged area also decreases blood flow. The heart has to pump harder against gravity if the injured area is raised to a level higher than the heart. At the same time, gravity will help any fluid that has accumulated at the injury site to move back toward your torso.

RICE also helps prevent any further injury. Rest avoids complications caused by moving the injured part. Ice prevents more bleeding, which can cause calcium deposits to form later. Compression helps support the injury. Elevation prevents you from putting any weight on the injured part, which could damage it more.

NOTE HOW THE INJURY HAPPENED

One of the most helpful, yet often overlooked, ways to lessen the extent of an injury is to note how the injury happened. Swelling and pain will often mask the actual injury, and it may be difficult for the doctor to examine the injury by the time a player has been brought into the emergency room or doctor's office. You, your tennis partner, or a coach should be able to say what you were doing at the time of injury. Often, using this information, I can make a precise diagnosis without being able to do a total physical examination.

USE THE RIGHT PAINKILLERS

I suggest three types of painkilling pills for my patients. I find these drugs to be valuable because they allow me to start aggressive, early rehabilitation of injuries.

Aspirin is the oldest and probably most widely prescribed drug. It not only kills pain but also reduces inflammation. The major side effect of aspirin is stomach upset and even bleeding from the lining of the stomach. If you have problems with regular aspirin, use buffered or enteric-coated aspirin instead. Another downside is that aspirin also interferes with blood clotting, so avoid it if you have bleeding injuries.

Acetaminophen pills, such as Tylenol, have the same painkilling effects as aspirin in most people, but do not have as much of an anti-inflammatory effect. They are less irritating to the stomach and have no anti-clotting effect. However, large doses can lead to liver problems.

Ibuprofen is the ingredient in nonsteroidal anti-inflammatory agents such as Advil. The various over-the-counter preparations are half-strength versions of the prescription medications. They all have a very strong anti-inflammatory effect and also have pain-relieving properties.

Anti-inflammatories must be taken carefully. They can have severe gastrointestinal (GI) side effects; they may irritate the stomach and cause bleeding, as well as ulcers. They can interfere with the production of the coating that protects the stomach and intestine from stomach acid. Anyone with a history of GI problems should not take anti-inflammatory agents, including those sold in drugstores, except under a doctor's direction. The doctor may prescribe accompanying medication to ameliorate the side effects.

When I suggest that tennis players take a painkiller, I let them choose whichever one they like the best. Most people know from previous experience which drug works well for them.

The only caveat is not to take aspirin along with anti-inflammatory agents. Since these two are chemically similar, adding one to the other could lead to a toxic reaction. So, for example, if you are taking ibuprofen for sore muscles and you get a headache, take Tylenol instead of aspirin.

USE FIRST AID FOR COMMON MUSCLE INJURIES

How to Treat Muscle Pulls

No matter how diligently you warm up and stretch, warm down and stretch, you may still pull a muscle from overuse, fatigue, or injury. A muscle pull is probably the most common sports injury after a bruise, one that you can do little, if anything, to prevent.

A muscle pulls when a sudden, severe force is applied to the muscle and the fibers are stretched beyond their capacity. If most of the fibers are overstretched and a few are torn, you have a muscle pull. If most of the fibers tear, it becomes a muscle tear.

The universally held treatment for a muscle pull or tear is to apply ice. This relaxes the muscle and helps relieve any spasm. Apply ice to the injured body part and rest it until the pain and swelling subside. You should apply the ice for about 20 minutes at a time for several days to reduce inflammation. Then you can start rehabilitating the body part with a gentle exercise and stretching program.

It is of the utmost importance to stretch the muscle while it heals. A pulled muscle usually goes into spasm, which is a protective mechanism that causes the stretched muscle fibers to contract. If the fibers are not gradually relengthened, the muscle will pull again once you return to activity because it will have healed in a shortened state. If you stretch the healing muscle gradually, not violently, you'll decrease your chances of reinjuring it.

In general, you can return to action when you are able to stretch the injured body part without pain as far as you can stretch the healthy one on the other side of the body.

How to Treat Muscle Spasms

If you show up on Monday at your doctor's office complaining of a "pulled muscle" from a weekend of tennis, you may have a delayed muscle spasm, not torn muscle fibers. Most muscle injuries cause some degree of muscle spasm or tightness. In fact, many mild muscle pulls actually end up in low-grade spasms. If you are not sure when the muscle began to hurt, you probably have not torn the muscle.

Some doctors like to give painkillers or anti-inflammatory agents as soon as possible after a muscle spasm starts, and suggest that you rest. Painkillers help prevent truly torn muscles from going into spasm. However, rather than keep my patients out of action with total rest, I prefer to get them involved in a gradual exercise program that uses a combination of icing and stretching.

First, apply a large cold pack to the muscle to numb it. A good way to do this is to make an ice cone by freezing water in a styrofoam cup, then peeling down the rim and rubbing the muscle with the ice until it is numb.

Next, start moving the sore muscle until you begin to feel tightness or pain. When the pain disappears, hold the injured body part in that position for a 20-second static stretch. A few moments later, contract the muscle slowly but fully, and hold for about 5 seconds. This isometric contraction will relax the muscle more.

Now move the body part again until you feel tightness or pain. Hold the body part for 10 seconds and then contract the muscle for 5 seconds. Repeat the stretch and contraction again, and then stretch the muscle one last time.

Let the body part rest naturally for 20 seconds, and repeat the entire program. You may need to renumb the muscle again between sessions.

This method of icing and stretching can also be used initially in muscle pulls and tears.

Within two or three days, the dull ache of the muscle spasm will be partially relieved. Then you can gradually resume full activities.

How to Treat Sore Muscles

Delayed muscle soreness and pain typically occur a day or two after strenuous exercise. The soreness usually subsides by itself within a few days. Mild exercise and liniment may help relieve the soreness.

Most athletes have used liniment to relieve the aches and pains of exercise. The unmistakable smell of liniment prevades locker rooms. I have found a direct correlation between an athlete's age, the ambient temperature, and the amount of smell—the older the player and lower the temperature, the worse the liniment smells.

Almost all professional teams use various balms on injured players, but sports doctors don't fully understand how liniments work. It's difficult to say whether liniment is directly responsible for an athlete's quick recovery and return to action. The actual massaging action of rubbing in the liniment, working it into muscles, may relax the muscle.

There are two basic types of liniments you can buy in a drugstore. The first includes Ben-Gay and Sports Creme, which typically contain menthol and methyl salicylate, an aspirinlike chemical. When you rub it in, your skin becomes slightly irritated, which causes an increase in blood flow to the area. This also produces heat, which relaxes stiff muscles. These rubs may also allow some salicylate to enter the bloodstream. Since salicylate is the active ingredient in aspirin, they may also have some pain-relieving effect.

The second type of rub, including Hot-Stuff and Atomic Bomb, depends on a substance called capsicum, which is the active ingredient in jalapeño peppers. An extract of this chemical is now being used as a prescription and over-the-counter ointment for arthritis pain, which is an indication that these rubs really do work. These hotter rubs have a much stronger irritating effect on the skin to stimulate blood flow. They give off so much heat that you can actually burn yourself, especially if you have fair skin. Go slowly when you use them until you can see how your skin reacts.

In addition to its use as an exercise rub, liniment is touted by some manufacturers as a warm-up aid. Liniment can help relax tight muscles and increase circulation. It may help shorten your warm-up time, particularly in cold weather, and may help maintain an increased blood flow after warm-down to reduce the lactic acid residue.

But don't think that because you have applied liniment that you are warmed up. A proper warm-up raises overall body temperature, not just the temperature in one muscle group. Think of liniment as a passive warm-up for one body part. Combine it with 10 minutes of light exercise, followed by stretching, to warm up the whole body.

Aspirin may also be helpful to relieve muscle soreness after a tough workout. Most weight lifters have sore muscles for a day or two after working out, and then the soreness disappears. This soreness often dissuades people new to strength training from going back to the gym for another session. Anti-inflammatory drugs, such as aspirin, may be able to ameliorate this discomfort somewhat. Several studies have found that taking aspirin after exercise reduces muscle soreness and improves the athlete's range of motion a day or two later.

For additional first-aid tips, look for this symbol throughout the book:

Medical Risks

Besides injuries, tennis players are subject to other medical problems related to the game. The previous chapter gave you specific advice about how to provide basic first aid. This chapter looks at other risks to your health and how to deal with them, including:

- Body heat problems.
- Sun exposure.
- Respiratory problems.
- Physical and mental burnout.

BODY HEAT PROBLEMS

The body has three cooling mechanisms: radiation, convection, and evaporation.

Radiation depends on the ability of the body to emit heat. As your body temperature rises, the small blood vessels (capillaries) in the skin dilate. This is why your skin turns red. Large quantities of blood rise to the skin surface where heat can be radiated to the outside to cool off the body. This increase in blood flow to the skin allows the heat to dissipate. However, exercising muscles demand large quantities of blood to supply oxygen and fuel. This reduces the amount of blood available to the skin, so radiation becomes less effective.

Convection depends upon the difference between your body temperature and the air temperature to transfer heat from the body. As the air temperature rises toward normal body temperature, the temperature difference decreases, and less heat is drawn off the body. So convection becomes less effective as the weather gets hotter.

Evaporation is the best source of heat loss. The evaporation of sweat is a cooling process. The higher the temperature, the more the body responds by increasing sweating. But high humidity interferes with this process: more moisture in the air means less sweat evaporates. With no evaporation, there is no cooling. So playing tennis on a humid day may be more dangerous than on a hot one. Also, if you keep perspiring without replacing body fluids, you become dehydrated. Excessive sweating leads to loss of body salts and potassium, which are collectively known as electrolytes.

What you wear can improve the effectiveness of your body's cooling mechanisms. The more skin exposed to the air, the more heat you allow to leave your body through the skin. Natural fibers transmit heat and allow evaporation better than artificial fibers. Light clothes reflect external heat better than dark clothes, so there is an advantage to traditional tennis whites on a hot day. Covering the body with clothing that does not provide good heat conduction can be dangerous and lead to heat exhaustion or heatstroke.

Tennis players have a choice to make on a hot, humid day. Exposing as much of the body as possible allows you to handle the heat better, yet covering up as much as possible helps avoid exposure to the sun. If possible, wear a wide-brimmed or long-peaked hat; lightweight, light-colored cotton shorts; a short-sleeved shirt; and short socks during the dog days of summer, along with plenty of sunscreen.

Heat Exhaustion

Heat exhaustion is due to dehydration and the loss of electrolytes. It causes you to feel light-headed and dizzy, and you may even faint. Your cooling mechanisms are working overtime, so you are sweaty and your skin is cool and clammy. You may also have severe muscle cramps due to the loss of salt and potassium. If you experience these symptoms, stop playing or practicing, rest in a cool place, and replace your fluids with water or an electrolyte drink, such as Gatorade. In severe cases, you may need to have fluids and electrolytes replaced intravenously at a hospital emergency room.

EMERGENCY *Heatstroke*

Heatstroke is a true medical emergency. In this case, all of the heat mechanisms have failed, and the body temperature has risen to the point where the brain's regulating mechanism has been knocked out. Body temperatures may go as high as 107 to 109°F. The symptoms of heatstroke are red, hot skin; lack of sweating; and, usually, loss of consciousness. Get someone with heatstroke to the emergency room immediately, where an ice bath, ice packs, or a cooling blanket can be used to help lower the body temperature. Someone with heatstroke could die very quickly without treatment.

Preventing Heat Problems

You can prevent heat problems by watching the weather and your fluid intake. In hot weather, you may lose up to one-half gallon of sweat per hour while on the court.

Check the temperature and humidity before you go out to play. If the temperature and humidity are both high, wait until they have both gone down, or simply cut down your playing time. Try to play early in the morning or in the evening, when temperatures are generally lower. Take a break in the shade whenever possible.

You need to begin drinking fluids approximately one hour before you play. To keep fluid intake up, take frequent water breaks, at least every 15 minutes, if not every changeover. Carry a bottle filled with plain water or an electrolyte drink, such as Gatorade, onto the court and leave it on the sideline in a cooler. Do not take salt tablets. They cause the body to extract large amounts of water to dilute the excess salt, which only causes more dehydration in the muscles. Continue to drink extra fluids for one hour after you come off the court.

Sports drinks contain all of the electrolytes plus fluid and glucose you need to replenish your energy. In a high-energy output sport like tennis, I recommend having 8 ounces of a sports drink at each set break. Water will do at changeovers. A sports drink is also helpful after a match to replace fluids.

SUN EXPOSURE

The sun's radiation has strengthened in recent years as the earth's protective atmospheric ozone layer has thinned. Heedless of warnings about exposure to the sun and the cancer risk it poses, millions of tennis players go out without protective clothing or sunscreens. But the risk of skin cancer should give any tennis player pause before heading for the court. The sun also affects the eyes, and sunglasses are a must on bright, sunny days.

What You Need to Know About Skin Cancer

About one in six Americans will have skin cancer, and about 1 million new cases are diagnosed each year. The most common types of skin cancer are directly related to sun exposure, which puts tennis players at risk because they spend so much time in the sun.

There are three types of skin cancer: squamous cell cancer, basal cell cancer, and malignant melanoma. Skin cancer usually is a culmination of many years of exposure to the sun. It is more common in fair-skinned people, who have a low pigment content in their skin. Sun damage is permanent, and just one blistering sunburn before the age of 20 doubles the risk of skin cancer for the rest of your life.

Squamous cell cancer and basal cell cancer usually appear as a persistent pimple or ulcer that will not heal. The skin may crust over, but it will open again. Squamous cell cancer is more common on the ear and lower lip, but may spread throughout the body. Basal cell cancer is most common on exposed areas of the skin and is not likely to spread, but it can be very destructive to the skin. If caught early, virtually all squamous cell cancers and basal cell cancers are curable with surgical removal.

Malignant melanoma is an aggressive skin cancer that may occur anywhere, but usually appears on an exposed surface of the body. It can spread to other body parts, where it usually is lethal. Signs of melanoma include an unusual-looking black mole that suddenly appears, or a persistent mole that suddenly enlarges.

Unless diagnosed early on and widely removed, melanoma can be rapidly fatal. Traces of melanoma may lie dormant in someone who had had a skin tumor removed, and then crop up decades later. About four in five people who have a melanoma removed from their skin survive another 10 years without a recurrence.

Melanoma is increasing in sunny regions that have large white populations, such as the U.S. Southwest. Between 1980 and the mid-1990s, the incidence of melanoma in the United States has doubled. More than

40,000 people are diagnosed with melanoma each year. Although regular skin examinations have saved many lives, more than 7,300 Americans die from melanoma each year. So it's important that you take precautions and see a doctor if you notice any changes in your skin.

Who is at Risk?

If you have more than 20 moles or a family history of skin cancer, you may want to see a dermatologist for regular checkups. If you live in a hot, sunny climate, more ultraviolet rays may reach your skin, and make you more susceptible to skin cancer. Melanoma may occur more frequently in those who have occasional, intense sun exposure.

There are signs you can watch for. These include new or changing spots, especially those that are asymmetrical, have irregular borders or bumpy surfaces, vary in color, or are larger than a pencil eraser. I recommend that every tennis player do a careful self-examination of his or her entire body before and after the season to detect any changes in existing moles.

Preventing Skin Cancer

Protective clothing and liberal use of sunscreens are very important, particularly if you play tennis several times a week. Anyone who plays in a climate with a strong tropical sun should take proper precautions.

A broad-brimmed hat protects the back of the neck and ears, which are highly susceptible areas. Darker clothes and hats block more dangerous ultraviolet rays than light-colored ones, but you have to balance out heat problems. A light-colored, cotton tennis shirt has a sun protection factor (SPF) of about 8.

A sunscreen takes 20 to 30 minutes to begin working, so apply it at least 30 minutes before heading outside. Wear a sunscreen that has an SPF of at least 15, and if you are out in the sun for more than one hour, reapply the sunscreen because you will be sweating on the court. (The SPF, incidentally, tells you how long the product is expected to protect your skin from burning. For example, a 15 SPF sunscreen should protect your skin from developing redness 15 times longer than no sunscreen at all. However, the reality is that thorough, frequent application of sunscreen is as important as the SPF rating.) The lips are especially vulnerable to sunburn, so use special lip sunscreens as well. Waterproof spray sunscreens work well for tennis players because they cover the skin quickly and don't leave your hands greasy.

Selecting a Sunscreen

Each person's need for sunscreen is different, depending on skin type and the duration of time spent in the sun. Selecting the proper product doesn't have to be confusing despite all the different SPF numbers on the labels and a dizzying array of ingredients. Each of the products is a little different, so it might take a bit of experimentation to find the product that is best for you.

If you follow simple instructions, using sunscreen correctly is easy. Here are some suggestions:

• Apply sunscreen thoroughly and evenly. The average adult needs about 2 tablespoons spread evenly over the entire body.

• Don't agonize over the SPF number. Most people should use an SPF of 15 if their skin is normal, or an SPF of 30 if they are taking photosensitizing medications (such as certain blood pressure pills) or suffering from a disease (such as lupus) that would make their skin unusually susceptible to burns. SPF numbers lower than 15 probably won't offer enough protection, while those higher than 30 may not offer any additional benefits.

• Buy a waterproof sunscreen. It won't be washed off as quickly by your own sweat, and so is useful even if you're not going swimming.

• Check the label to make sure your sunscreen protects against both ultraviolet A (UVA) and ultraviolet B (UVB) light since sunlight contains both types of ultraviolet rays.

• Be alert for sunscreen allergies, which may show up as rashes. If you have a skin reaction, switch to a brand with different ingredients. Generally, sunblocks with titanium dioxide are less likely to cause allergic skin reactions. Most sunblocks work by absorbing light, but the "physical" sunblocks, such as titanium dioxide, work by reflecting and scattering the sun's rays. Also, the fragrance or preservatives in a sunscreen can cause irritation, so simply changing brands (regardless of active ingredients) can sometimes be effective.

• If you are extremely sensitive to sunlight, use zinc oxide or an equivalent sunblock that keeps out all light. You no longer have to live with that white, pasty look with the introduction of new zinc sunblocks that come in fluorescent colors. Also, both antibiotics and Retin-A make your skin more sensitive to the sun and increase the chances of a sunburn. So if you are using these medications, make sure to apply lots of sunscreen.

Eye Problems

Tennis players need to wear sunglasses for the same reason they apply sunscreen: harmful ultraviolet light can also affect the eyes. Ultraviolet light levels are typically higher from late spring through the summer, which is the peak tennis season.

Sunlight that reflects off the court can burn cells on the eye's surface. A few years of sun exposure can cause unsightly, fleshy growths called pterygiums on the whites of the eyes. Usually harmless, they sometimes spread over the iris and interfere with vision.

A lifetime of playing tennis without eye protection increases your risk for some serious ailments. Over the years, ultraviolet rays damage the eye's lens. Proteins in the lens may clump together to form brown or milky clouds known as cataracts. Lens surgery can often restore vision loss caused by cataracts.

Cataracts are known to occur more frequently in tropical or sunny climates. Prolonged exposure to sunlight is definitely a risk factor in the formation of cataracts. The definitive study was conducted on fishermen in the Chesapeake Bay area over a 20-year period. The fishermen who wore sunglasses had a much lower incidence of cataracts than those who did not. The Johns Hopkins researchers who conducted the study advise wearing a hat with a brim and close-fitting sunglasses with ultraviolet-absorbing lenses at times of maximal exposure to sunlight.

Ultraviolet light may also injure the macula, an area of the eye that enables you to see fine detail. If lesions form, a condition called macular degeneration, this type of sharp vision is irretrievably lost.

Protecting Your Eyes

Good sunglasses help keep your eyes healthy. The lenses should block at least 99 percent of ultraviolet rays. The color or tint of the lenses is unimportant as long as they block ultraviolet rays. A polarized lens will also reduce glare off the sand or grass. Wraparound or large-frame glasses block more light, and wraparounds prevent light from seeping in from the sides.

A handful of manufacturers, including Bolle, Carrera, and Gargoyles, now make sunglasses specifically designed for tennis. These sunglasses are generally lightweight, shatter-resistant, and adjustable, and offer distortion-free lenses that keep out the wind, dust, and glare.

Most of them have interchangeable lenses with different tints. The most common lens tints include gray and green, which make colors appear as they are, but do not help depth perception; amber and yellow, which enhance depth perception but distort color, and are best used in low-light conditions; and brown and copper, which combine true colors and good contrast. The sunglasses cost about $100, with additional lenses going for $25 to $45. In general, these glasses are comfortable to wear even during a long match, can enhance court vision, and protect your eyes from harmful ultraviolet rays.

Incidentally, while eye injuries are not common in tennis, they tend to be the most severe of any sport. Sunglasses with a sturdy frame and unbreakable lenses provide some protection from being struck in the eye with a tennis ball.

Eye-care companies are also marketing new contact lenses that block harmful ultraviolet light. These extended-wear contacts, coated with ultraviolet-absorbing chemicals, block up to 90 percent of ultraviolet rays and cost about the same as normal contacts. Like wraparound sunglasses, they do not let light in from the sides.

RESPIRATORY PROBLEMS

Allergens can cause problems such as allergies and asthma, which can affect your breathing and your game.

Allergy

Being an outdoor activity, tennis raises the potential health problem of allergies. Tennis players are at risk by their exposure to allergens, and I don't just mean those who play on grass courts. Nasal allergies affect about 35 million Americans, and the effects can be debilitating. The symptoms include sneezing, allergic rhinitis, itchy, tearing eyes, and swollen eyelids. If you have a cold that lasts longer than a week to a week-and-a-half, the chances are you have allergies.

In people with allergies, the body mistakes allergens such as pollen, wood products, dust, and animal dander as enemies that need to be destroyed. When the body attacks these allergens, your nose becomes inflamed and swollen. This inflammation causes the nasal allergy symptoms.

One way to control allergies is to control their causes. This means avoiding or eliminating allergens that may trigger an allergy attack at home and at work.

Most people with allergies can control bothersome symptoms with drug therapy. For some, over-the-counter antihistamines, decongestants, or nasal sprays are effective. Others require prescription medications. It may be necessary to experiment under the guidance of a physician to determine what the most effective medication is for you.

Since allergy pills take about one hour to work, they should be taken before you start to play. Nasal sprays work within minutes, but you might need to take them again while on the court, so I recommend that tennis players take the longer-acting oral allergy preparations.

Asthma

Asthma is a chronic, sometimes fatal disease in which allergens or irritants inflame airways in the lungs, which can close up suddenly and impair the ability to breathe. The most important substances or conditions that trigger asthma are allergies, upper respiratory infections, cigarette smoking, secondhand smoke, dust, cold air, exercise, aspirin, and air that contains particles, sulfur dioxide, ozone, or smog.

Most asthma seen among tennis players is due to allergies. Asthma attacks may also be induced by exercise, usually within the first 5 to 10 minutes. About 70 percent of the 15 million Americans with asthma wheeze and cough when they exercise or when exposed to allergens. About 10 percent of the population has exercise-induced asthma.

Mild symptoms can be managed by reducing the intensity of exercise or with the help of an inhaler. To prevent an attack, I recommend a slow, prolonged warm-up of at least 15 minutes and a longer, but slightly less vigorous playing time. An inhaler can be used before playing, if necessary. Also make sure that someone else knows the location of the inhaler and whom to call in case of an emergency.

Tennis players with exercise-induced asthma can exercise safely by using the same bronchodilating drugs prescribed for asthmas of other origins. In many cases, physical conditions can reduce symptoms of exercise-induced asthma. Sports with periodic rests, like tennis, are less likely to cause attacks than a continuous activity, like jogging.

Since all asthma drugs are by prescription, a physician should help you decide which preparations would be best for you and oversee your treatment. Asthma should not prevent anyone from playing tennis since it is very manageable with modern drugs.

PHYSICAL AND MENTAL BURNOUT

When you constantly train at the high end of your target heart rate, you risk problems with fatigue, muscle injury, and stress. Trying to work out like an elite athlete can run you into the ground.

"No pain, no gain" is not the best way to condition yourself. Fatigue and injuries can result from pushing yourself too hard. You will find that you can achieve better results by cutting back on your exercise and tennis intensity. Your body and mind need to rest and recuperate. Backing off training just before a big event lets your muscle strength and stamina increase.

High-intensity training may also counteract the good feelings you get from playing tennis. Tennis is a great way to reduce stress and anxiety and to lift moods. But long training sessions may actually make you feel more tense, depressed, and angry. The symptoms of overtraining include fatigue, insomnia, irritability, and soreness and a normal workout that seems harder than usual.

Mental Aspects

Almost all sports are based on competition. Even the recreational tennis player will at times try to attain his or her personal best and play a little harder. Striving to reach peak performance is fine until you push yourself past your capacity. This usually occurs at the end of a match, when your muscles are tired and more prone to injury.

Working Through an Injury

Many tennis players refuse to take time off because of their drive to keep pushing themselves. I often hear a tennis player say, "I laid off for three days when I pulled a hamstring, but it didn't get better." It can be difficult to get the message across that a hamstring pull may take three weeks to heal. The tennis player just doesn't want to hear it.

And once treatment begins, I inevitably hear, "Do I have to stop, or can I keep playing?" This mental outlook often interferes with even the best treatment because the tennis player will try to play before he or she is ready. Listen to your doctor and your body and let any injuries recover properly.

Health Gadgets

Tennis players are always looking for an edge. Like many sports, tennis has become more competitive, even for casual players. Players who may have once played a few friendly sets on the weekend now end up competing in weeknight leagues and club, or even national amateur, championships. They will do anything, and try anything, to be able to beat the pants off their partners the next time out.

This eagerness to get better at almost any cost makes tennis players vulnerable to health gadgets that may or may not have any value. Some are so far on the fringe of medicine that they smack of quackery. Others have some validity when used properly. Here's a look at what works, and what doesn't, among the current collection of health-related items marketed to tennis players.

BRACES

Tennis Elbow Braces

Tennis elbow is the bane of any tennis player's existence. In addition to an exercise program (see chapter 9), tennis players can use a variety of counterforce braces to protect against this all-too-common injury. From bands to a single bar to double bars, these braces compress the extensor muscle in the arm and help relieve the elbow pain. One of the best is the Air Cast, an inflatable brace that not only can help control pain but prevent recurrences.

Knee Braces

With the advent of minimal knee surgery, more tennis players are able to continue to enjoy the game by wearing a variety of stabilizing knee braces. The new braces are ideal for arthritis, cartilage damage, and instability problems. Some you simply wrap around and attach with Velcro closures. Others have flexible side stays to add support, plus an opening behind the knee to eliminate pinching and binding. Still others "unload" the knee—that is, take a load of weight off the knee—with a plastic brace that attaches both above and below the knee.

If you have knee problems, ask your doctor which type of brace is best for your particular problem, and then test out a few different models for comfort and support.

Ankle Braces

Air Cast also makes an inflatable ankle brace. Anyone who has recently sprained an ankle is at high risk for a recurrence until the ankle heals completely. Inadvertently stepping on a tennis ball may result in your ankle turning over again, forcing you to go through another painful ankle rehabilitation (see chapter 14). The Air Cast brace, worn on top of your tennis shoe and over the ankle, prevents the ankle from turning over. At the same time, it may limit your ability to get around the court quickly.

Other ankle supports provide overall compression and protection with nonbulky designs. Some use elastic with Velcro straps, while others use leather with laces. These fully adjustable braces allow you to control the fit and level of support you need. They fit comfortably over all shoes for hours of tennis.

Back Braces

Low-back pain is also a common problem among tennis players. A variety of back-bracing products are available to provide added back support and relieve muscle pain and stress. They sell for about $60 at tennis shops or through catalogs.

The Tourbelt looks like the back brace worn by construction workers or heavy weight lifters, except that it has an inflatable air bag in the back pack. A valve allows you to pump as much or as little air into the belt as needed. This varies the amount of support to your lower back. The belt can be worn under or over your tennis clothes.

Solid S'port is a pair of elastic shorts with an adjustable, elastic, built-in, low-back support. Two tapered side pulls distribute support throughout the lower back. The manufacturer claims the fabric wicks away moisture, but it appears that it might be uncomfortable on a hot day.

Any back support is helpful for a tennis player with low-back pain, but I do not recommend them to prevent back troubles. Constantly using back braces prevents back muscles from strengthening themselves because the support does all of the work, not the muscles. The muscles become dependent on the support and end up more prone to injury.

MAGNETS

In the early 1980s, I received a set of medicinal magnets to test. Since my wife, Gail, had a bad foot at the time, I put the hard, metal piece in her shoe. The salesman insisted it would help her, but it only made her foot feel worse. He also gave us a large metal magnet to put under our mattress to reduce my back pain. "You'll feel one hundred percent better when you get out of bed," he said. The only thing it did was make me sleep with my head pointing north.

Medicinal magnets have been around for more than a dozen years with claims of relieving back pain, tendinitis, arthritis, and headaches. While professional athletes claim that wearing magnets helps relieve back pain and has allowed them to return to top form, there has been no medical evidence to show that magnets have any effect on athletes. In part because of endorsements by professional athletes, Americans now spend large sums on magnets for pain relief. The Food and Drug Administration has warned manufacturers and doctors about health claims for magnets.

Magnets theoretically stimulate nerve endings, which may help restore energy and increase blood circulation. The most popular ones are a series of small magnets worn in a belt around the back, which is supposed to relieve lower-back pain, sciatica, and muscle stiffness, and to increase range of motion, which is essential for tennis players. Other magnets inserted into insoles are designed for tired, aching feet, bunions, heel spurs, and arthritic conditions, and into knee and elbow sleeves and wrist wraps to combine support and compression with magnetic therapy.

These small magnets marketed to tennis players cannot be very potent. The amount of magnetic force generated by these small magnets is very little.

There is something to be said for the idea of suggestibility. If a tennis player thinks the magnet is going to work, it may well work some. Since there is little evidence that magnets do anything, the only way to explain pain relief is through the placebo effect. The placebo effect comes from controlled, scientific studies in which neither the doctor nor the patient know whether the medication the patient is taking is real or a dummy pill, known as a placebo. This type of study allows researchers to see whether a medication is really effective compared to the placebo, which theoretically should have no effect. In fact, medical studies show that if a doctor tells patients they are taking medicine, and gives them sugar pills, up to 40 percent of those patients will actually respond to the placebo.

Although the exact source of a placebo's power is unknown, experts attribute it to mind-body interaction. They suspect it may be linked to the hope and belief that the substance will work. By taking it, the person may be aware that he or she is doing something to help control his or her condition. When people have a strong belief in a treatment, it changes their natural pain mediators and endorphins, the substances that boost the body's natural ability to tolerate pain.

Spontaneous relief of symptoms does occur, although rarely. If enough people use magnets for pain relief, a few will likely feel better.

Over the years, I have tried small magnets a number of times with New York Giants players because I had heard anecdotes of pain improvement from athletes and trainers. I have never found any improvement in symptoms or healing time over standard therapies. Since I have never heard a player say, "Yes, I feel better using magnets," I have discontinued using them.

There is a place in sports medicine for high-potency electromagnets to stimulate healing of hard-to-heal fractures. These magnets may be imbedded in a cast or strapped onto a limb. The high-energy electromagnetic field has been shown to improve healing in certain cases. These magnetic fields are much more potent than the small magnets sold to tennis players.

Copper Bracelets

Professional tennis players were among the first to endorse copper bracelets back in the 1960s. A wide variety of claims for improvement of arthritis, tendinitis, and assorted aches and pains have been made for thin, copper bracelets worn around the wrist. The theory is that these conditions may be due to copper deficiency and that small amounts of copper are absorbed through the skin from the bracelet.

There has never been any reproducible scientific evidence that these bracelets are effective. Some people do seem to feel better, again possibly through suggestibility and the placebo effect. The results are usually temporary and do not actually treat the underlying problem. That is significant for people with progressive diseases, such as some types of arthritis. In general, arthritis patients need something that actually slows down the destruction of the joints. While it's good that a placebo makes you feel better, it has no long-term impact on disease progression.

Since we know that copper bracelets don't cause any harm, there is no reason for tennis players who feel better to take the copper bracelets off. It may turn their skin green under the bracelet, but nothing else harmful will happen to them.

Alloy Bracelets

Another type of bracelet is made of a metal alloy and features a ball on either end of the wrist band. It supposedly corrects an imbalance in positive and negative energy. I'm not quite sure what positive and negative energies are and how they get out of balance. Nowhere in medical literature or human physiology are these energies discussed. Eastern medicine touches on balancing out the chi (also spelled qi), or energy throughout the body, but I believe this is more metaphysics than medicine. I would place alloy bracelets in the realm of snake oil.

FOOD FADS

High-Energy Bars

High-energy bars are basically beefed up granola bars. They contain about 200 calories, many more than simple granola bars. Energy bars are really designed for high-output workouts like tennis. They probably are useful for tennis players to overcome hunger and will definitely help improve energy levels, particularly if a match or practice lasts for longer than one hour. The small packets are certainly easy to carry and quick to eat.

Experiment during practice to see which energy bars your stomach can tolerate and which ones taste the best. Drink at least 16 ounces of water with each bar to aid digestion and to help keep your fluid level up.

Sports Nutrition Gels

Sports nutrition gels concentrate a high amount of energy into a gel pack that is swallowed, not chewed. These gels contain many more carbohydrates than the same amount of a sports drink.

Chewing can be difficult during high-intensity exercise, such as tennis, but I still don't recommend these gels. Stick with a sports drink and high-energy snack, and drink water at every changeover.

TENNIS RACQUET PROPERTIES

Keeping up with technological advances in tennis racquets can be difficult. Things change rapidly, and you have to be able to figure out which changes are based on scientific evidence and which ones are just marketing gimmicks.

The latest trend in racquets is less weight, thanks in part to the use of titanium or titanium/graphite composites. These lightweights weigh in at about 9 or 10 ounces—half that of many wooden racquets of the past. The advantage is a faster swing, better control, and more power, particularly for beginning to intermediate players with compact swings.

Other racquets have wider, stiffer frames, longer handles to extend your reach, and bigger hitting surfaces to improve your chances of hitting the ball. The trend is toward racquets that are more maneuverable, stable, and comfortable to hit.

Make sure to get the right head size for your game. A baseliner should opt for a racquet with a heavy head. A serve-and-volley or all-court player should go lighter. The new ultralong racquets can help baseliners reach more balls and serve-and-volleyers to contact the ball higher, which increases serving accuracy and reach on stretch volleys.

Use the largest grip that is comfortable. Today's grips can be smooth, spongy, perforated, ribbed, and treaded. The wrong grip size, or worn-out grips, can contribute to blisters.

Maximize your racquet's performance by altering the string type, thickness, and tension. Traditional gut strings add power and control but tend to break often. A slightly cheaper alternative is high-grade synthetic string. Or try a thinner synthetic string, which provides more power and control but will also break more quickly. Normally, strings wear out after about six months, or 30 to 40 hours of playing time.

Part Three

What to Know from Head to Toe

The Head and Neck

THE HEAD

While head injuries are not common in tennis, they do occur, particularly in doubles play where the bodies or racquets of two partners may come into contact.

✚ Bruises and Cuts

Bruises, or contusions, are usually caused by being hit by the ball on a smash. It's more common in doubles because the player at the net has less time to react. Being hit by your partner's racquet may also cause a bruise.

Bruises can usually be treated just by icing them to reduce swelling and to control pain. If the skin is broken, then clean it with soap and water and apply an antiseptic spray or cream. Aspirin or an anti-inflammatory may also help ease the pain faster.

Cuts, or lacerations, can also occur from being hit by your partner's racquet. If the cut is minimal, simply clean it with soap and water and coat it with an antiseptic or antibiotic cream. A severe cut should be sutured by a physician.

(EMERGENCY) Concussion

A concussion is any loss of consciousness, even for a moment, or disorientation after a blow to the head. This can happen from a hard blow from a racquet or from running into your partner. There are many degrees of concussion. A player may be unconscious for several minutes with a severe concussion. Another player may be stunned for a few seconds and have trouble remembering where he is or what he is doing.

If a blow causes loss of consciousness or memory or disorientation, the player should be seen by a physician.

The treatment for a concussion is to rest to protect against further injury to the head. If you immediately regain consciousness or are out for just a short time, someone should watch you carefully for signs of persistent headache, nausea, and further loss of consciousness. These are the danger signs of possible bleeding inside the head, and if they appear have someone else take you to a hospital as soon as possible for observation and a neurological examination. A typical neurological exam after a concussion will include checks on your reflexes, muscle strength, balance, and pressure in the back of your eye.

Broken Nose

A blow to the nose by a racquet or ball can fracture the nasal bones or the cartilage of the septum, the area dividing the two nostrils. A broken nose often is obvious: the nose appears to be flattened or crooked, there is lots of bleeding from the nose, and breathing is difficult.

Any nose suspected to be broken should be iced down to limit swelling and bruising. Then have the nose x-rayed and examined by a doctor. Once fixed, the nose should be protected with a splint until it heals completely, which can take four to six weeks.

MD Eye Injuries

Most eye injuries are caused by being struck in the eye with the tennis ball. Rarely, you may be hit by your partner's racquet.

Eye injuries may cause a bruise that looks like a black eye, scratch your cornea (the clear covering of the eye), cause bleeding inside the eye, or even cause a detached retina. Any injury to the eye should be seen immediately by an ophthalmologist. A scratched cornea is usually an extremely painful—though minor—injury. But if severe, and not cared for, it can lead to loss of vision. Cover the eye with a patch and see a doctor as soon as possible.

Direct blows to the eye from a tennis ball can be prevented. To protect your eyes, you can wear protective eye gear, especially if you have already had an eye injury. Every eye injury must be considered serious. Sight is one of our most precious gifts and should be protected at all times. Again, cover the eye and get to a doctor.

🆙 *Blowout Fracture*

A blow to the eye or cheek from the racquet can fracture the bones surrounding the eyeball, called the orbit. A blowout fracture is easy to spot: since the orbit connects to one of the sinuses, when the victim blows hard through the nose, the eye will suddenly swell shut as air gets into the tissues right under the eye.

As with any fracture, the victim of a blowout must see a doctor for treatment, which may include surgery.

THE NECK

Along with the head, the neck is the area affected in most of the serious injuries I see. The neck is much less stable and much more prone to injury than the rest of the spine. At the top of the spinal column, the vertebrae in the neck become progressively smaller. The neck is tremendously mobile in order to allow the head to swivel, so the range of motion between the vertebrae in the neck must be greater than in the lower spine. Also, neck muscles are much weaker than those in the lower back, where the strongest muscles in the body support the spine.

🆙 *Pinched Nerve*

An injury that seems like a sprain but is more complex is a pinched nerve. This happens when a cervical disc ruptures or degenerates. Commonly, when a disc ruptures, jellylike material from inside the disc presses on a nearby nerve and causes sharp pain that extends down into your arm. You may feel a sudden onset of severe pain in your neck, or the pain may come on slowly over time.

Tennis players, who may make fairly violent neck motions, are prone to pinched nerves. A pinched nerve usually responds to some form of cervical traction (neck brace) for two to six weeks, with accompanying physical therapy to reduce muscle spasm. However, if severe symptoms persist, particularly in the arm and the hand, you may need surgery to repair damage to the disc.

✚ Neck Muscle Injuries

When you wake up in the morning and can turn your head only one way, you are suffering from wryneck, or spastic torticollis, which is due to a pulled muscle or muscle spasm. The same type of injury can happen when you look up and serve or hit an overhead smash. Or your neck may be stiff due to overstress. You feel the pain on one side of the neck, and your neck may be pulled over slightly to that side. It's particularly painful to turn your head in the direction of the pain. That is, if the pain is on the left side of your neck, you can turn to the right but not to the left.

The proper treatment is to apply ice for 20 minutes at a time and gently stretch the neck (see the exercises on the following page). If the pain is severe, you may need medication, such as a muscle relaxant or anti-inflammatory agent, and physical therapy.

✚ Trapezius Triggers

Severe muscle spasm in a localized area of the neck can cause another injury, called triggers of the trapezius, characterized by a very painful area at the base of the neck or extending out above the collarbone. Any tennis player can incur this injury by pulling fibers in the trapezius muscle or suffering a direct blow to the muscle fibers in the neck from a ball or racquet.

The muscle spasm in the neck sets up a reflex arc that feeds on itself. The spasm causes nerves to fire and gives the sensation of pain. The electrical impulse causes other nerve fibers to fire and the muscle to contract more. This, in turn, causes the pain fibers to fire, starting the cycle all over again.

For treatment, ice the neck for 20 minutes and massage it gently with your fingers while stretching the muscle (see Trapezius Stretch, page 74).

If the pain is severe, you may need physical therapy, including electrotherapy, which involves electrical stimulation of the neck muscles. Very severe pain may require an injection of cortisone or novocaine.

Preventing Neck Injuries

Probably the best way to prevent a neck injury is to strengthen your neck muscles. The huge necks on football players do not happen by accident. They are a result of long hours of exercise to increase neck muscle strength.

Every tennis player should work on improving neck strength. You can do basic exercises by applying resistance against yourself or by working with a partner.

Neck-Strengthening Exercises

Neck Tilt against Resistance

Tilt your head to the right while applying resistance with your right hand, or have a partner apply resistance. Hold for 20 seconds. Then tilt your head to the left and resist with your left hand for 20 seconds. Do the same exercise tilting your head forward and backward.

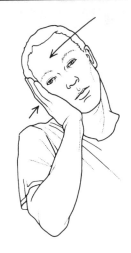

Shoulder Shrug with Barbell

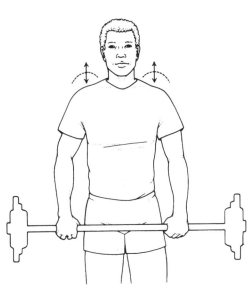

Hold a barbell with 50 to 100 pounds of weight straight down in front of you with your elbows locked. Now shrug your shoulders and hold for 5 seconds. Do five repetitions for five sets. This helps build up the trapezius muscle in your neck. If you are starting out, you may need to use less weight and build up gradually to the specified weight.

A Stretching Program for Pain Relief

To help alleviate minor neck pain, here are some simple exercises. Probably the best stretch of them all is the Trapezius Stretch. If you have serious neck problems, consult your physician before trying these exercises.

Neck-Stretching Exercises

Trapezius Stretch

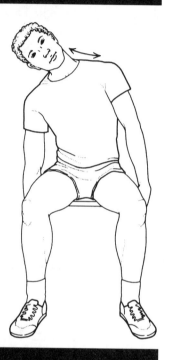

Sit in a chair and hold onto the seat with the hand of the painful side. Now bend your trunk and your head to the opposite side.

Funky Pigeon

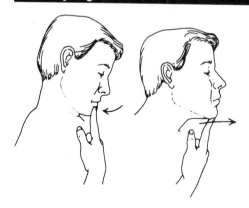

While sitting down, look slowly to the side, first over one shoulder, and then over the other, five times back and forth. Then get "funky" like a pigeon: jut your chin forward and back five times.

Shoulder Shrug

Lift both shoulders up to your ears and then drop them as low as they can go. Do this five times.

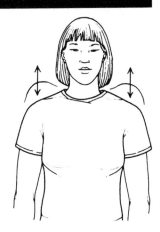

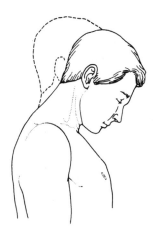

Chin Drop

Gently drop your chin to your chest. Now move your chin in a semicircle from shoulder to shoulder five times.

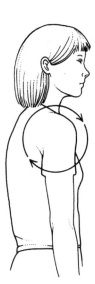

Shoulder Roll

Roll your shoulders by making a circle. Lift both shoulders and roll them forward five times, and then lift and roll them backward five times.

7

The Shoulder

The shoulder is one of the most often injured joints among tennis players, particularly among junior elite players. The shoulder is a unique joint and is extremely prone to a great many injuries. It's a very shallow ball-and-socket joint. The head, which has little contact with the small socket, can easily slide out of the socket, which means that the joint is not very stable. The rest of the shoulder socket is formed by ligaments that connect various parts of the bony components of the socket, and cartilage around the small rim of the bony socket.

The shoulder is the only joint in the body not held together by ligaments. The few ligaments in the shoulder only serve to keep the shoulder from moving too far in any one direction. The ligaments have little to do with holding the joint in place.

The shoulder socket also contains three tendons: the tendons of the long and short heads of the biceps muscle and the supraspinatus tendon. The biceps tendons connect the biceps muscle to the bones of the shoulder and help the biceps flex the forearm. The supraspinatus tendon connects the supraspinatus muscle and the bone of the shoulder, and aids the supraspinatus to move the humerus, the bone between the shoulder and the elbow. Directly below the socket is the brachial plexus, which houses all of the nerves that supply the arm.

The shoulder bones are held together by a group of muscles you read about all the time on the sports pages: the rotator cuff muscles. These muscles are responsible for the shoulder's fine movements, such as hitting a serve. Because of the shoulder's shallow socket and lack of ligaments, any weakness of the small rotator cuff muscles makes it easy for the head of the shoulder to slide partway out of the joint, which is a partial dislocation or subluxation. Or it may slide all the way out, which is a full dislocation.

ROTATOR CUFF INJURY

Sports in which you bring your arm up over your head, such as tennis, are the main contributors to overuse injuries of the shoulder. The rotator cuff muscles are not meant to function under any stress with the arm above parallel to the ground. If the shoulder joint is continually stressed with the arm in this overhead position, the small rotator cuff muscles begin to stretch out. This allows the head of the joint to become loose within the shoulder socket.

If the head of the shoulder is loose, it will slide forward when you extend your arm backward over your shoulder, catching the tendon of the short head of the biceps between the ball and the socket. The same thing happens if you raise your arm to the side so that it's higher than parallel to the ground. The head will drop in the socket, and the tendon of the long head of the biceps becomes impinged. The supraspinatus muscle may also become impinged.

The impingement causes the nerves under the shoulder to fire and shoot pain down through the tendons of the shoulder into their connecting muscles. Tennis players feel the pain particularly in the long head of the biceps. Tennis players with this injury always tell me they can hit their ground strokes effortlessly, but when they try to hit an overhead or serve, their shoulder hurts.

How Not *to Treat Rotator Cuff Problems*

Many doctors overlook the true problem with a shoulder impingement. They treat the tendinitis (inflamed tendons) with anti-inflammatory agents or cortisone (steroid) injections. But the anti-inflammatories soon wear off, and the next time you hit a serve, the tendon will be pinched or impinged upon again. The pain returns, requiring another injection or more anti-inflammatories.

All too often, I have seen a high school or college tennis player with a sore shoulder whose doctor tells him not to play for a while, just to rest it. So he rests it and the pain subsides. But as soon as he returns to playing, the pain returns. He has wasted his rest time and now must stop playing again until he has properly corrected the problem.

The Correct Treatment for Rotator Cuff Injuries

The proper way to treat a shoulder impingement is through an exercise program to strengthen the rotator cuff muscles sufficiently so that the head of the shoulder is held firmly in place and will not slip out of the socket. With no slipping, the tendons will no longer be inflamed or irritated.

Rotator Cuff Strengthening Exercises

You can re-strengthen your rotator cuff muscles initially at home with a free weight program. Using 15 pounds as the absolute maximum weight, do the following exercises until fatigue sets in, or 50 repetitions once a day:

Arm Curl

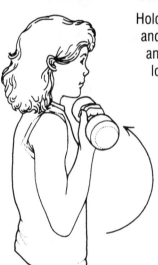

Hold a dumbbell with your palm facing forward and your hand at your side. Bend your elbow and lift the weight to your shoulder. Slowly lower the weight to the starting position.

Reverse Arm Curl

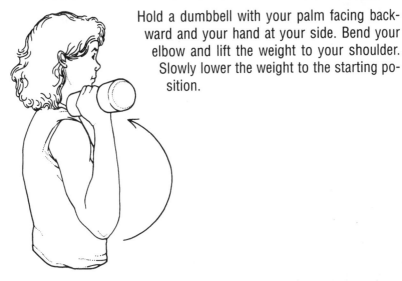

Hold a dumbbell with your palm facing backward and your hand at your side. Bend your elbow and lift the weight to your shoulder. Slowly lower the weight to the starting position.

Front Lift (Palm Up)

Hold a dumbbell at your side, palm facing forward with elbow locked. Lift the weight straight up, but no more than parallel to the floor. Slowly lower the weight to the starting position.

Front Lift (Palm Down)

Hold a dumbbell at your side, palm facing backward with elbow locked. Lift the weight straight up, with your arm no higher than parallel to the floor. Slowly lower the weight to the starting position.

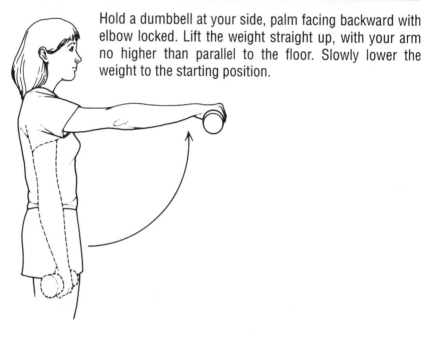

Lateral Lift

Hold a dumbbell at your side, palm facing the body. Lift the weight to the side, with your arm no higher than parallel to the floor. Slowly lower the weight to the starting position.

Bent-over Lateral Lift

Stand and bend over at a 90° angle. Grasp a dumbbell and, with elbow locked, lift the weight straight up to the side. Again, go no higher than parallel to the floor. Slowly lower the weight to the starting position.

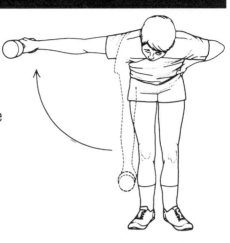

Bent-over Chest Lift

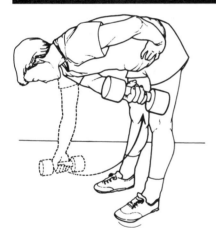

Stand and bend over at a 90° angle. Grasp a dumbbell and, with elbow locked, lift the weight across your chest. Slowly lower the weight to the starting position.

Your doctor may prescribe physical therapy, in which case a physical therapist can design an exercise program for you. Three out of every four rotator cuff problems can be cured with simple exercises.

If the problem has not begun to disappear in six to eight weeks, then you may need to use special isokinetic exercise machines, such as Cybex machines. These machines use a computerized system that senses your effort and, at any given millisecond, adjusts the resistance to meet your force. Also, some movements of the shoulder, such as the follow-through after a serve, are hard to rehabilitate with free weights. Unless you stand on your head, the weight is coming down by the force of gravity and offers no resistance. A Cybex machine provides the proper resistance for any motion.

Some people do not respond to rehabilitation, even with physical therapy, and will require surgery to repair the shoulder joint.

A ROTATOR CUFF TEAR

A torn rotator cuff used to mean the end of weekend tennis matches. Tearing these muscles left the shoulder weak. Today, tearing the rotator cuff muscles is not as big a problem because of better rehabilitation programs and much better surgery.

A torn rotator cuff receives the same initial treatment as a stretched one—a good rehabilitation program. The surgery is difficult and should be avoided, if at all possible. Consider surgery only if you don't respond well to rehabilitation.

If the tear is not too large, a simpler surgery through a lighted tube, or arthroscope, may be possible. Arthroscopic surgery, which has revolutionized treatment of the knee, is coming into more widespread use for the shoulder. Repairing the rotator cuff muscles through the arthroscope provides a new, less invasive way to treat this injury.

Another potential problem with a rotator cuff tear develops during the recovery period after surgery. When you rest a shoulder, as you must for four to six weeks after rotator cuff surgery, and avoid moving it in certain ways, the shoulder loses its ability to make those movements. The result may be a partially frozen shoulder with limited motion. This requires a diligent rehabilitation program, and it can be a long, painful process to get the shoulder to move through its full range of motion.

✚ 🅜🅓 SHOULDER MUSCLE PULLS

Like any area of the body, the shoulder is subject to muscle pulls. The mechanism is the same: the muscle overcontracts or overstretches, causing muscle fibers to tear. Typically, I see this among tennis players.

The proper treatment is a short rest period, about three to seven days, followed by stretching and then strengthening exercises. As with all muscle pulls, you should warm up and then stretch and lengthen the shoulder muscles to prevent pulling them again.

Because of the complexity and number of muscles around the shoulder that can pull, you need to see a physician to get a diagnosis of which muscles are involved and a physical therapist for a program specifically designed for those muscles. You cannot rehabilitate torn shoulder muscles yourself. Find out which ones are torn and what to do for them.

✚ MUSCLE IMBALANCE

The repetitive demands of tennis place the shoulder under maximum stress. Often, tennis players are not able to limit the load placed on their shoulder muscles the way baseball pitchers do by limiting their number of pitches or the frequency of pitching.

Maintaining adequate strength and muscle balance may be a factor in preventing shoulder injuries. The strength and power of the muscles that accelerate the arm during the serving motion, called the internal rotators, tend to become strong in tennis players, particularly among younger elite players. The opposite muscles, the external rotators, which help decelerate the arm in the serving motion, do not increase proportionally in strength. This creates a functional muscle imbalance that may lead to an overload of the external rotators and subsequently to shoulder muscle injuries. Exercises that strengthen the shoulder in external rotation (see below) will help maintain a favorable muscle balance, and may prevent or lessen the severity of these injuries.

External Rotator Muscle Strengthening

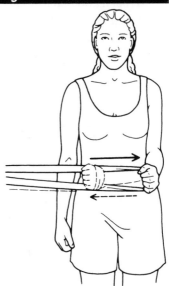

Tie a 4-foot-long piece of rubber tubing or a similar length of TheraBand to a doorknob. Stand a few feet away from the door, with your hips perpendicular to the door. Wrap the other end of the tubing or band around your right hand (for right-handers) and pull your hand across your body until it reaches your right hip. Keep your elbow close to the body throughout the motion. Work your way up to three sets of 8 to 10 repetitions. You can shorten the tubing or band to increase resistance.

〔MD〕 THE OTHER SHOULDER PAIN: BURSITIS

Some doctors call any kind of shoulder pain "bursitis." However, true bursitis only occurs in the pillowlike sacs of fluid, called bursa, found throughout the body. These sacs vary tremendously, from the size of a lemon pit to that of a large lemon. Bursas occur where a tendon has to turn a corner and go around a bone. They allow the tendon to slide freely without wearing itself out when rubbing against the bone. Overstressing these little sacs causes them to become inflamed. Once they swell up, they become extremely painful.

Bursitis is different from tendinitis, although both can be very painful. Usually, you don't feel the pain of tendinitis unless you use the tender body part. With bursitis, the body part is painful whether you move it or not. Also, you feel the tenderness of tendinitis all along the length of the tendon, but you feel it in one specific spot with bursitis.

The treatment for bursitis is usually a cortisone injection. You may have heard horror stories about your next door neighbor having an injection for bursitis and how painful it is. Unfortunately, most of those stories are true. Putting more fluid into an already inflamed sac causes a flare-up of severe pain for about a day. Once the cortisone takes effect, however, it cools down the inflammation, and the pain subsides.

I have found that the more humane way to treat bursitis is with cortisone by mouth for the first few days. The pills almost always provide rapid relief, and in many cases, the bursitis calms down completely without any need for injections. Some bursitis sufferers, however, may still need injections because of the discomfort. These later injections do not cause the same amount of pain since the inflammation and swelling in the bursa have already been reduced.

✚ SHOULDER POPS: PARTIAL DISLOCATION

A sudden force exerted against the shoulder can also cause the head to slip momentarily out of the socket—that is, become partially dislocated, or subluxated. The shoulder's structures and shallow socket may allow the head to slip partway up onto the rim of the socket, and then the shoulder snaps back into place spontaneously. It feels as if your shoulder has "popped" out and then "popped" back in. But that's not really what happens. If the shoulder was truly dislocated, with the head all of the way out of the socket, then it wouldn't pop back in spontaneously. Most people can't put a dislocated shoulder back in place by themselves. Often, it's difficult for an experienced physician to get it back in place.

When the shoulder head slides partially out and then snaps back in, it stretches the rotator cuff muscles, and you have the same problem as an overuse injury. The shoulder begins to slide around, causing an impingement and tendinitis. Because the rotator cuff muscles are stretched, the head is more likely to slide out again. The rotator cuff gets looser and looser until finally your shoulder is in danger of truly dislocating.

The standard treatment for a subluxated shoulder is rest. But that's not enough. Your resting shoulder may not hurt, but the rotator cuff muscles are not getting any stronger. If the muscles stay loose, then the shoulder joint can still slip later on. You must use the same exercises described earlier to strengthen the rotator cuff muscles to prevent future slipping.

These muscles are slow healers. The strengthening program usually takes 6 to 12 weeks, and the shoulder may not be back to full strength for six months or more.

✚ FULL DISLOCATION

A shoulder becomes fully dislocated when the head comes all of the way out of the socket. This requires a much greater force than that needed for a partial dislocation.

A dislocation may stretch or tear the rotator cuff muscles. Usually, these muscles are just stretched, particularly among younger tennis players. Older tennis players, who have more brittle rotator cuffs, are more likely to tear the muscles.

When I first started practicing sports medicine, the standard treatment was to immobilize a dislocated shoulder for six weeks. But even after six weeks, the shoulder never really worked well again, so we cut the immobilization time to three weeks. Now we know that rest is effective only when the rotator cuff muscles are also restrengthened. I can't emphasize enough that if you have shoulder pain or discomfort, even though it will go away with rest, you must restrengthen your rotator cuff muscles through an exercise program to regain full use of your shoulder.

It used to be that two shoulder dislocations meant surgery. And without rehabilitation after the first dislocation, the second one happened quite frequently. Today, even with multiple dislocations, a good rehabilitation program can often tighten the shoulder muscles so that no surgery is necessary.

✚ SHOULDER SEPARATION

Separation of the acromioclavicular joint, where the end of collarbone meets the shoulder blade, is actually a sprain of the ligaments that connect the two bones. "Separation" is an old medical term that has been applied to the widening of the space between the bones. Since this problem involves ligaments, it really should be called a sprain.

As with all sprains, there are three degrees of severity. A mild, or first-degree, sprain causes a minimal stretching of the ligaments without much tearing of fibers, and the joint remains stable. There will be pain and swelling around the joint.

In a moderate, or second-degree, sprain, the ligaments are stretched more and partially torn, and the outer end of the collarbone will partially snap in and out of the joint. I diagnose this type of sprain by first taking an X ray of both shoulders. Then I have my patient hold a 25-pound weight in each hand and take another X ray. As the weight pulls the two bones apart, the joint of the affected shoulder will be visibly wider on the second X ray.

It's much easier to diagnose a severe, or third-degree, sprain. The complete disruption of all of the ligaments around the joint causes the collarbone to stand straight up in the air.

The primary cause of a shoulder separation is falling on the point of the elbow, which drives the shoulder up.

The treatment for first- and second-degree shoulder sprains is rest. You will have to put the shoulder in a sling for one to three weeks, depending on the severity of the injury. Also, in addition to resting the shoulder, you must ice it for 20 to 30 minutes a few times a day in the beginning to ease the pain. These are particularly frustrating injuries because they can take six to eight weeks to heal. You will not be able to raise your arm laterally above 90° until the injury has healed.

For a third-degree shoulder sprain, surgical repair of the ligaments is necessary to fix the joint. Up to six weeks of recovery from surgery are necessary before you can begin a restrengthening program. This program consists of range-of-motion and strengthening exercises similar to those used to rehabilitate a shoulder impingement.

The Back and Ribs

COMMON BACK PROBLEMS

Even though the back muscles are the strongest in the body—you can lift four times as much weight with the back than you can with the arms and shoulders—a tennis player with weak back muscles will likely have back problems. Nearly all injuries to the back are muscular in nature. About 95 percent of low-back pain is the result of muscular problems caused by a lack of exercise, weak muscles, or being overweight.

Most tennis players have more well-developed back muscles on the dominant side (right side for right-handers). Back problems can be due to weak or tense muscles or muscle strain from suddenly overloading these muscles during activity. Muscle fibers will pull or tear, sending the back muscles into spasm and causing pain.

Fortunately, most simple backaches go away within a few weeks, with or without treatment, and 90 percent of them disappear within two months. A tennis player who works out to strengthen the lower back and abdominal muscles may be able to prevent back pain.

The greatest stress on the back is from the serve and, to a lesser extent, from overheads. The spine in the back hyperextends and rotates while you rotate your hitting shoulder away from the net on the toss. The trunk then powerfully flexes to the side. Then your hitting shoulder and trunk rotate toward the net as you flex forward.

A traditional forehand has you rotate your body 90°. An open-stance forehand has less rotation, but the acceleration is greater. A one-handed backhand involves less trunk rotation than a forehand. A two-handed backhand has more rotation and places the spine in the back at risk, particularly when you reach for a wide ball.

✚ Back Spasm

The sudden twists, turns, and lunges associated with tennis may cause back muscles to become irritated, to pull, and eventually go into spasm. When back muscles go into spasm, the force is so great that you may be disabled by the excruciating pain. When these muscles go into spasm and shorten, it can cause your back to tilt severely to one side.

The treatment for back spasm is rest for a few days, medication such as aspirin or other anti-inflammatory agents, and possibly muscle relaxants. Use ice for as long as you feel pain. You may also need support from a girdle and physical therapy, which starts with ice, then heat, electrical stimulation of muscles, stretching, and deep massage to relax the muscle. This should be followed by an exercise program to strengthen the back, described later in this chapter.

Disc Problems

Discs are the fibrous pillows filled with a gel-like material found between the vertebrae. They act as shock absorbers for the spine, cushioning the vertebrae as they move against each other.

Tennis players are at a somewhat high risk of developing disc disease because of the quick, repetitive, rotational movements. However, most back pain is muscular.

MD Bulging Disc

One of the most common back problems is a bulging disc. The wall of the disc bulges out into the spinal column. The disc, however, is not ruptured completely.

The disc bulge looks like a weak spot in the inner tube of a tire. The pressure of this bulge on the spinal cord or on the nerve roots coming out of the spine causes the pain. However, many people with bulging discs have no symptoms at all. The diagnosis can only be made by a magnetic resonance image (MRI), so see your doctor for treatment. Treatment usually consists of rest until the symptoms disappear.

MD *Ruptured Disc*

A ruptured, or slipped, disc usually occurs in the lower (lumbar) spine, the area that takes the brunt of twisting and turning. A lifetime of poor posture, lifting heavy objects, and repetitive twisting motions in tennis can weaken the discs and eventually cause a rupture.

A ruptured disc, also called a herniated disc, occurs when the disc capsule breaks open and protrudes into the spinal canal, pressing on nerve roots. Gel oozes out of the disc and causes more pressure on the spinal cord or the nerve roots. Over time, the gel usually disintegrates, and the symptoms are relieved.

When a disc ruptures, however, the pad between two connecting vertebrae is gone, and the gradual wearing of bone on bone leads to arthritis. This can cause serious pain if the arthritic spurs of the vertebrae press on the nerve root. The pain will worsen as years go by without treatment.

The pain of a ruptured disc is usually sharp and sudden. Commonly, the pain will be passed along the course of the nerve impinged by the ruptured disc. A disc pressing on the sciatic nerve root causes sciatica, sending pain from the buttock down the leg and into the foot.

A bulging disc cannot be seen on a normal X ray, but can be picked up easily on a computed tomography or MRI scan. Only when the disc has completely disintegrated can the narrowed space between two vertebrae be seen on X ray. So you may need more than a simple X ray for your doctor to make the correct diagnosis.

Many ruptured discs will respond to bed rest. When you stand, each disc carries the weight of the body above it. Therefore, you need to take the weight off the disc. Often, the disc will heal if you lie down until the pain recedes.

A back brace may help relieve the stress on the disc, and physical therapy can help relieve any muscle spasms associated with a ruptured disc. After you have passed that first stage of acute pain, you will need to engage in a back-strengthening program.

If your symptoms do not subside, you may need surgery to remove some or all of the disc. What used to be a crude, major operation with long disability has now become a much more sophisticated, simpler procedure with little difficulty afterward.

The majority of patients get better without surgery, even those with acutely ruptured discs. Surgery is prescribed for the 10 to 15 percent of patients who don't respond to conservative treatment or who feel a weakness or numbness in their limbs, which is a sign of neurological problems.

The classic back operation, called a discectomy, involves an incision in the lower back and removal of a small piece of the vertebra to expose the injured disc. Then the damaged part of the disc is cut out. Surgery now usually involves insertion of an arthroscope into the ruptured disc to suck out the gel and relieve the pressure on the nerve.

MD *Cracked Back*

A fracture of part of the vertebra connecting the front and rear portions of the bone is called spondylolysis. Originally, this was thought to be a congenital failure of the two halves of the vertebrae to fuse. Now we believe that this is due to acute fractures caused by back trauma.

I see spondylolysis most commonly among young people who have chronic, recurrent back pain for no good reason. Often, they have taken a fall before they report feeling any pain. A vertebra may also crack with a stress fracture from excessive movement in the spine, which is common in tennis due to the excessive twisting and turning.

If an X ray reveals a fractured bone, I have to decide whether the fracture is fresh or old. A bone scan, a simple nuclear medicine procedure, helps identify fresh activity in the bone.

If the fracture is old or congenital, the treatment of choice is a strengthening program with reduced physical activity until the symptoms cease. If the fracture is fresh, the patient must stop playing tennis for six months to see whether the fracture will heal. Usually, rest alone is not enough to relieve all the symptoms, and a program to strengthen the back muscles is required afterward.

A back brace may be helpful during this time. However, a brace should only be used when you feel acute pain. Back braces are not useful in the long run because they further weaken the back.

PREVENTING BACK PROBLEMS

The basic prevention for back problems is to develop a strong back. Since most injuries are due to muscle weakness or injury, increased strength is the answer to almost every back problem.

In the past, back doctors and sports medicine experts have always recommended exercises that strengthen the flexor muscles of the back.

This may be why back treatments have not been very successful. The flexor muscles of the back are the ones that pull the back forward and down. But the body is naturally pulled in that direction by gravity. To lift your trunk into an erect position, you must use the extensor muscles. These are the muscles that you need to strengthen. Once you get through early flexion exercises, you must concentrate on extension exercises.

Recognizing the need to concentrate on extensor muscles has led to a change in the philosophy on how to recondition an injured back. Also, working with machines such as the Cybex, we have found that we can work muscles beyond the point of pain. The machine will indicate when you have reached the danger point and should stop exercising.

Also, through the use of electromyograph (EMG) machines, which measure muscular activity, researchers have found that the traditional sit-up used to strengthen the abdominal muscles actually does more harm than good. The EMG results show that a sit-up with the fullest range of motion offers more potential for damage than a simple abdominal curl.

A Back-Strengthening Program

Back pain is never quite the same from one person to the next, and there are many different types of self-treatments. I prefer ice treatments for 20 to 30 minutes at a time two or three times a day for as long as the back is sore. I prescribe heat on the back only to loosen it up before activity once it has healed.

Bed rest for more than a couple of days only weakens your muscles and can be disabling. You need to get up out of bed as soon as possible. Surgery should be considered only as a last resort.

If you suffer a back problem, chances are you will wind up on a regimen of daily back-stretching and back-strengthening exercises to recondition your back. These exercises are designed to strengthen the muscles that support the back, especially the abdominal muscles; to stretch overly tight muscles and ligaments in the back so that they are less likely to be injured; and to reduce the defects in posture that strain the back. Strong, flexible muscles around the lower back and abdomen stabilize the spine and protect it from injury.

Back-Stretching and Flexion Exercises

You can do back exercises at home to strengthen both your extensor and flexor muscles. To strengthen an acutely injured back, you should start with stretching and flexion exercises.

Slow Toe-Touch

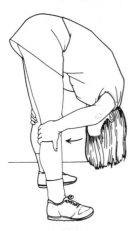

Lower your forehead between your knees while standing. Go as far as you can go, and then grasp behind your knees and try to go a little farther. Hold for 10 to 15 seconds. Slowly return your body to the starting position. Start with 3 repetitions and then increase gradually by one every second day until you reach 12 repetitions.

Toe-Touch with Rotation

Spread your legs and bend at the waist with your forehead in the direction of your right knee. Hold for 10 to 15 seconds. Slowly stand up straight again and then lower your forehead toward your left knee. Hold for 10 to 15 seconds. Start with 3 repetitions and then increase gradually by one every second day until you reach 12 repetitions.

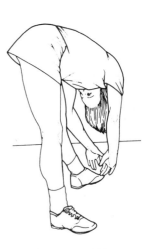

Hurdler Stretch (Standing)

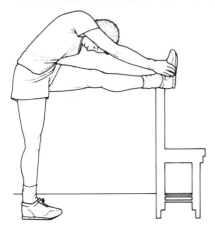

While standing, put one foot on a chair in front of you. Now bend your forehead forward and try to touch it to your knee. Use the same number of repetitions as for the toe-touch exercises. Repeat with the other leg.

Knee Pull with Head Curl

This exercise increases flexibility in the hip, lower back, and buttock muscles. Lie on your back with knees bent and feet flat on the floor. Bring one knee up toward your chest and clasp the knee with both hands. As you curl your head up, pull the knee down gently. Hold for 10 to 15 seconds. Return the leg to the starting position and do the same number of repetitions as for the toe touches. Repeat with the other leg.

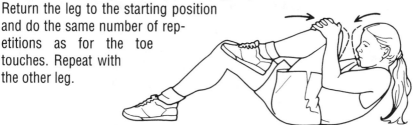

Pelvic Tilt

While lying on your back with knees bent and feet flat on the floor, relax the back muscles and tighten your abdominal muscles to press your back flat against the floor. This will tilt your pelvis forward. Once you have a totally flat back, do the same number of repetitions as for the toe touches.

Abdominal Curl

Lie on your back, knees bent and feet flat on the floor with your hands clasped behind your head. Slowly curl your shoulder blades up off the floor, leaving your back on the floor. Hold for 5 seconds, then slowly lower your head and shoulders. Start with five repetitions, increasing by five as the curls get easier.

Extension Exercises

As you become more comfortable and your back muscles begin to lengthen again, you can start extension exercises.

Back Extension

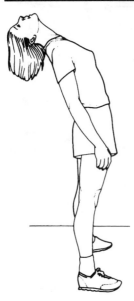

Stand up straight, arms at your side, and slowly lean your upper body back from the waist. Try to look at the ceiling. Hold for 10 seconds, then relax and straighten up. Do five repetitions and build up by twos as the stretch becomes easier.

Hip Extension

Lie on your back on a table with one leg hanging down over the side. Gently lower the leg from the hip towards the floor. When you feel the stretch in your hip, hold for 10 seconds. If possible, have a partner push on your knee to increase the stretch. Return your leg to table height and repeat the stretch five times. Add on stretches two at a time as this becomes easier.

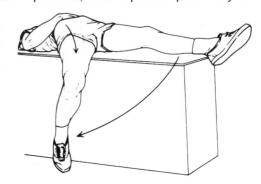

Reverse Sit-up

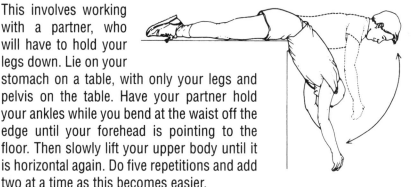

This involves working with a partner, who will have to hold your legs down. Lie on your stomach on a table, with only your legs and pelvis on the table. Have your partner hold your ankles while you bend at the waist off the edge until your forehead is pointing to the floor. Then slowly lift your upper body until it is horizontal again. Do five repetitions and add two at a time as this becomes easier.

Pain-Free Tennis

Orthopedists often advise back-pain sufferers to avoid sports that put severe stress on the back. However, a back problem should not doom you to a life of inactivity. You can continue to play tennis if you take some precautions.

Tennis can be challenging for anyone with back pain with all of its twisting, flexing, and extending motions. If you are plagued by a bad back, try to flatten out your serve to eliminate excessive arching and twisting. You may also consider wearing a back brace. Try to pick up balls by lifting them between a foot and the racquet rather than bending at the waist.

Many tennis players also show poor posture between breaks in the action. Tennis players spend more time waiting to exercise than they do actually participating in the sport. Try to maintain good posture before and after each point.

THE RIBS

The ribs are bones in the chest that attach to the vertebrae of the spine. There are 12 ribs on each side of the body. They perform two functions: they act like bars around a cage to protect the lungs and heart from blows; and they help the chest wall expand and collapse so that air can move through the lungs.

The ribs do not attach directly to the breastbone in the front. If they did, the rib cage would be so rigid that you would not be able to breathe. Flexible cartilage connects the end of each rib to the breastbone.

✚ *Pulled Muscle*

The muscle between each pair of ribs, the intercostal muscle, which is the muscle used in respiration, may pull or tear due to overstress. This can happen to a tennis player who makes a sudden, violent lateral motion or suddenly rotates the rib cage.

As a result, you will feel tenderness between the ribs, not on them. Rest the ribs and ice them until the pain disappears, and use anti-inflammatories, if necessary. An elastic wrap around the chest can help you move about freely. Since it is impossible to strengthen or stretch these muscles, you just have to wait for the pain to disappear before resuming play.

If the pain is more than mild, see a doctor to rule out a more serious injury such as a rib separation or fracture.

The Elbow

After 10 years away from the game, Jan returned to tennis when he moved to the suburbs with his wife and daughter. "I met a few guys who were at my level, and slowly began to get my game back," says the 40-year-old author, who had been the number one singles player on his high school tennis team. He began to play singles regularly on weekends, and also joined a top-level doubles game one night a week.

But all that tennis all at once put a strain on Jan's elbow. "I couldn't even pick up a racquet. I did the exercises Dr. Levy recommended, and within about a month, I was back playing." Now he's contending for the club championship in singles, and won the mixed doubles with his wife.

The elbow is an important joint for tennis players not only because of its varied uses, but also because it is a common source of misery. Tennis elbow is usually the main topic of conversation in most tennis clubs. About half of all tennis players suffer from tennis elbow during their playing days. Those in the 35- to 50-year-old age group are the most likely to complain of elbow pain.

You are five times more likely to feel pain on the outside of your elbow as on the inside. Factors that increase the chances of tennis elbow include increasing age, more frequent play, weakness and inflexibility in the forearm muscles, lack of foot movement, poor accuracy in hitting shots, and a too-tight grip on the racquet.

The elbow is actually three separate joints, consisting of the junction of the two bones of the forearm with each other and the junction of each of those bones with the humerus, the bone of the upper arm. These three interfaces allow the elbow to bend and straighten and also to rotate, which allows you to move your hand from palm up to palm down.

An elbow injury can be especially troubling because it can also be caused by wrist problems. The muscles that control the wrist originate from the elbow's bones. As a result, many of the problems that arise from excessive wrist strain cause pain in the elbow rather than the wrist.

✚ TENNIS ELBOW

The most common elbow injury in tennis is the proverbial tennis elbow. Tennis elbow is really an inflammation of the muscles of the forearm and the tendon that connects the muscles to the bones in the elbow. These muscles are used to bend the wrist backward and to turn the palm face up. When the muscles and tendon become inflamed from overuse, you feel pain on the outside of your elbow (the lateral epicondyle). The pain is worse when you try to lift things with your palm facing down, so you may have trouble picking up a coffee cup or taking a quart of milk out of the refrigerator.

Tennis elbow also causes pain when you rotate your hand in a clockwise direction, as you would in using a screwdriver to put in a screw or in screwing in a lightbulb. You also will feel pain when you clench or squeeze something, such as when you shake hands or hold a racquet. The pain may become so severe that it makes combing your hair virtually impossible.

A tennis player most often aggravates the elbow by hitting the ball late on the backhand swing. The backhand, most players' bête noire, is an especially difficult stroke to master. By hitting the ball with your weight on your back foot, you have to overcompensate by using mostly your arm, and hitting late causes your elbow to be bent. You end up straining the forearm muscles and tendon. You can also get tennis elbow by constantly turning your wrist to put more spin on the serve.

I often see tennis elbow when players try to step up in class and they find that the ball is coming at them harder. The elbow ends up absorbing most of this shock. Also, they may be a little late hitting the ball because of its speed.

Using old tennis balls, which have less spring off the racquet and put stress on the elbow, a heavy racquet, and weak forearm muscles can all contribute to tennis elbow.

Treatment for Tennis Elbow

Once your elbow becomes inflamed, everyday activities are enough to keep it irritated. Giving up your weekly tennis game to rest your elbow is not enough to solve the problem. Treating tennis elbow requires an exercise program to increase the strength and flexibility of the forearm muscles and tendon. Once they are strong enough to withstand the stress of a bad backhand, then the pain will go away and won't return.

If you have a history of tennis elbow or feel twinges of pain after playing, wait at least half an hour after your match and then ice the elbow down. Icing is more effective once the elbow has returned to normal body temperature. I usually tell my patients to apply ice as soon as they get home. Fill a plastic bag with a mixture of ice and water, and keep the elbow cool for up to 30 to 40 minutes.

Forearm-Strengthening Exercises

You will need a small dumbbell—5 pounds for men and 2.5 pounds for women. The weight can be gradually increased as your strength improves.

In addition to the strengthening exercises shown here, do Arm Curls (see page 78) and Reverse Arm Curls (see page 79).

Wrist Curl

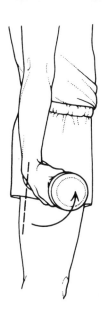

Hold the dumbbell with your arm down by your side and your elbow locked. With your palm facing forward, flex the wrist forward all the way and then let it back down. Repeat 50 times or until the muscle is exhausted.

Reverse Wrist Curl

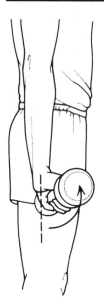

Put your arm down by your side and turn your hand so that the palm faces backward. Holding the dumbbell, flex your wrist forward as far as it will go and then let it down. Repeat 50 times or to the point of muscle exhaustion.

Unbalanced Wrist Rotation

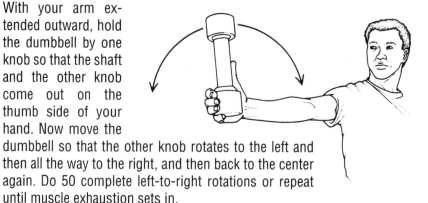

With your arm extended outward, hold the dumbbell by one knob so that the shaft and the other knob come out on the thumb side of your hand. Now move the dumbbell so that the other knob rotates to the left and then all the way to the right, and then back to the center again. Do 50 complete left-to-right rotations or repeat until muscle exhaustion sets in.

Roll-up

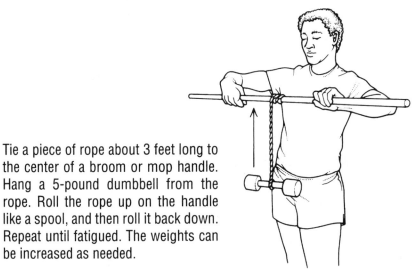

Tie a piece of rope about 3 feet long to the center of a broom or mop handle. Hang a 5-pound dumbbell from the rope. Roll the rope up on the handle like a spool, and then roll it back down. Repeat until fatigued. The weights can be increased as needed.

Ball Squeezing

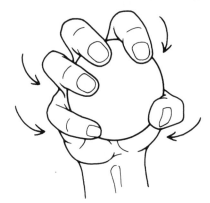

Hold a soft, rubber ball and squeeze it continually until your hand is fatigued. Sporting goods stores also carry a substance called hand putty, which can be used in the same way.

Elbow Flexibility Exercises

When you start the exercise program, you may feel some pain because you are overloading the elbow to make it stronger. The following flexibility exercises will help relieve this pain.

In a week to 10 days you should begin to feel better. You may need to use anti-inflammatory agents during those first 10 days of therapy.

Elbow Stretch (Palm Up)

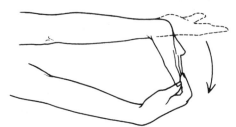

Extend your arm straight out, parallel to the floor, with the elbow locked, palm facing up. With your other hand, push the palm and fingers of the extended hand toward the floor. Hold for 15 to 20 seconds.

Elbow Stretch (Palm Down)

Extend your arm straight out, parallel to the floor, with the elbow locked, palm facing down. Push the top of your hand and fingers of the extended hand down toward the floor with your other hand. Hold for 15 to 20 seconds.

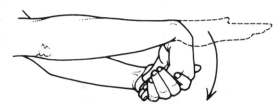

"Just Say No" to Cortisone

In the past, and even now, the standard treatment for tennis elbow has been cortisone injections. This is definitely *not* the best long-term treatment. Injecting an anti-inflammatory agent, such as cortisone, around an inflamed tendon will reduce the inflammation and ease the pain. But this doesn't address the cause of the problem, which is overstressing the forearm tendon.

When the cortisone begins to wear off in four to six weeks, the forces that caused the tendinitis in the first place will remain, causing the pain and stress to recur, and you will need a second injection of cortisone. To remain pain-free, you will have to repeat the whole process again and again. This may be good for your doctor's bank account, but it isn't good for your elbow. Eventually, these cortisone injections can irreparably damage the tendon.

Other Options

Occasionally, I have patients who are resistant to an exercise program. I then use a cortisone injection to reduce the inflammation so that they can actively work on strengthening the elbow without too much pain. I use cortisone only as a last resort, not as a primary treatment for tennis elbow. I also put some patients into physical therapy, where they can exercise under supervision.

I may also introduce deep friction massage. This is a quite painful technique in which a physical therapist applies deep thumb pressure back and forth across the tendon. The irritation causes increased blood flow to the tendon and promotes healing. Another way of increasing blood flow is with electrotherapy, which passes an electric current through the tendon.

Another treatment is iontophoresis, in which a cortisone solution is painted on the skin and then driven through to the tendon by way of an electric current. This concentrates cortisone around the tendon without subjecting the tendon to the damage of an injection.

Every one to two years, I have a patient who needs surgery to repair a tennis elbow. This rare patient has detached some tendon fibers from the bone and has a dead spot in the center of the tendon. The only therapy is surgery to clean out the dead area of tendon and then to reimplant the tendon.

Alternative Treatments

The World Health Organization lists 104 conditions that are treatable by acupuncture, including tennis elbow. Acupuncture involves inserting thin needles into various points in the body. This is said to help correct and rebalance chi (or qi), which Chinese medicine believes is the body's vital energy.

Acupuncture treatments work for about two out of three tennis elbow sufferers. It usually takes two to five visits to a licensed acupuncturist. An appointment typically lasts between 30 and 60 minutes and costs about $50 to $100. Check to see whether your insurance company will pay for the treatment.

No one knows why acupuncture works for some and not for others, but some believe it is due to endorphins, the body's natural painkillers. I believe it has to do with the placebo effect—if you believe a treatment works, it will have a much better chance of working. If you don't feel noticeable pain relief in three or four visits to an acupuncturist, then it probably isn't worth your while to continue.

Another alternative treatment—injections of botulinum toxin, which causes botulism—is now being used by researchers in the Netherlands in cases of chronic tennis elbow. Botulinum injections have become a popular method for smoothing facial wrinkles by temporarily paralyzing the muscles that tug at the skin. But I don't see how this would work for tennis elbow, and recommend running the other way if someone suggests you try it.

How to Prevent Tennis Elbow

To prevent tennis elbow, do the same strengthening and flexibility exercises that were outlined for treatment. Also, make sure that you warm up and stretch your arm before playing a vigorous set. You should also seek the advice of a tennis instructor to correct your backhand stroke so that you hit the ball properly. Power your serve and backhand with your legs, body, and shoulders, not your wrist and forearm. Beginners should learn a two-handed backhand stroke, which is less likely to cause tennis elbow because you generate more power by using both arms and turning your body more.

Wearing an elbow band, either a single or double band with a bar, is definitely beneficial for tennis elbow. These counterforce braces compress the muscles and reduce the shock transmitted to the tendon. Clinical studies show that these braces act as a cinching belt. They short-circuit the force of the muscle contraction, particularly in the serve and backhand drives.

A counterforce brace contains a nonelastic, padded girdle that fits the contour of the forearm. It is held in place by two small buckles and Velcro straps. It functions as a constraint against muscle contraction and excessive movement of the tendons. This reduces the force and overload on the soft tissues of the elbow.

When a muscle contracts, it tends to expand. The counterforce brace controls the expansion and reduces the forces developed by the muscle. The brace, however, won't interfere with your game because it does not prevent motion.

Another type of counterforce brace is the Air-Cast band, which is also nonelastic, but contains an air bubble. This brace also has been shown to be effective at reducing muscle activity.

You can get a counterforce brace through your physician or sporting goods store. Don't strap your brace too tightly. You should feel its pressure only when the forearm muscle contracts and expands.

Choosing the proper tennis racquet and string pressure can also prevent tennis elbow. Tennis elbow sufferers should use a composite or graphite racquet since these transmit the least amount of shock to the elbow. (The old wooden racquets, alas, were the best in lessening the shock.) The racquet should be strung loosely and should be no larger than midsize. An oversized racquet not only has a bigger sweet spot in the center but also a much larger, elbow-shocking hitting area around the rim. Also, hitting out on the rim of an oversized racquet is a shot you probably would have missed with a smaller racquet, which would have spared your elbow.

Manufacturers are now producing lighter, stronger tennis racquets with increased padding to enhance the racquet's shock-absorbing abilities. The new light titanium racquets, when used with a damper, have significant power with no annoying vibration shooting up the arm.

Lower your string tension to dampen shock—usually 3 to 5 pounds less than the manufacturer's low-range suggestion. Higher string tension does give more control, but also increases the shock to your arm after ball impact. A multifilament, high-grade synthetic string also provides a softer string bed to reduce vibrations to your racquet. You may want to try one of the new racquets with double strings that claim to reduce the shock transmitted to the arm.

An increased grip size can also help. Too small a grip can lead to arm muscle fatigue from overtightening. A tight grip on the racquet transmits vibrations to the hand and arm. Cushion grips can also help decrease the vibration transferred to your forearm. Elite players and those with good technique can benefit from tightly gripping the racquet. Casual, recreational players will save themselves from injury by using a loose grip on the racquet.

Play on slower surfaces, such as clay or Har-Tru, which absorb some of the impact from the ball. Always follow through with your backhand stroke since stopping short places stress on the elbow tendons.

✚ Tennis Elbow II

Another type of tennis elbow causes pain on the inner side of the elbow (the medial epicondyle). This pain involves inflammation of the muscles and tendon that allow you to pronate the wrist—that is, turn the wrist over so that the palm faces down. I see this elbow pain in tennis players who hit topspin forehands, which require them to turn the racquet head over the top of the ball. Many top-ranked tennis players feel pain on the inner side of the elbow because they hit a lot of topspin shots. For the weekend player, the culprit may be a late forehand that requires snapping the wrist and pronating the forearm.

Prevention and treatment measures are the same as for the other type of tennis elbow. The exercises outlined earlier also strengthen and stretch the inner side of the elbow. I also recommend that you work on your swing mechanics with a coach.

✚ TORN BICEPS

A sudden, severe movement of the arm can tear the biceps muscle. One head of the biceps can be literally torn in half. This is usually seen in an older tennis player who hits a hard forehand smash. The torn muscle causes pain, bleeding, loss of function, and muscle deformity.

You need to take care while recovering from a biceps tear. If the biceps contracts as the swelling subsides the upper part of the muscle can ball up, causing a defect the size of a small orange on top of the muscle.

Cosmetic surgery can correct the muscle defect, but it cannot bring the muscle back to its original strength. The buildup of scar tissue weakens the muscle. In fact, a torn biceps muscle that has been repaired will likely tear again.

Treatment involves allowing the torn muscle to rest for two or three weeks while it heals. This is followed by a training program to strengthen the other head of the biceps so that it can take over full function of the muscle. Arm Curls are the best exercise to strengthen the biceps muscles (see page 78).

10

The Wrist and Hand

THE WRIST

The wrist is one of the more complex structures in the body. There are 10 bones involved in moving the wrist joint in multiple directions. These include the 2 forearm bones and 8 other small bones. These small bones are extremely sensitive to excessive force or trauma, such as that generated in snapping the wrist in tennis, which makes the wrist one of the more frequently injured parts of the body.

✚ SPRAINED WRIST

The most common injury to the wrist is a sprain. With all of the stresses the wrist is subjected to in tennis, there is a good chance that the ligaments interconnecting the wrist bones will be sprained. Many people also have weak wrists because there are few muscles in the wrist to stabilize it.

All but the most minor wrist sprains should be x-rayed because of the possibility that a sprained ligament may pull off a little piece of bone, which changes the injury to a fracture. A sprained wrist may not need anything more than a soft splint. A fractured wrist, however, requires casting.

The treatment of a sprained wrist, as for any sprain, is immediate immobilization, rest, and ice, then a set of range-of-motion exercises followed by strengthening exercises. Use the same exercises outlined in chapter 9. These same exercises help take the pressure off the wrists to help prevent injuries. An elastic wrist support may also be helpful.

The ultimate wrist sprain is a subluxation of the wrist bones. This happens when the ligaments connecting two or more of the small bones become completely torn and the bones slide out of place. Ageless tennis ace Jimmy Connors had to have his wrist completely rebuilt surgically after years of overuse. The long, arduous rehabilitation from surgery requires the services of a good hand therapist for the tennis player to regain full motion of his or her wrist.

MD *Broken Wrist*

Any severe wrist pain following a fall or blow to the wrist should be seen by a physician and x-rayed because of the possibility of a fracture. One or both of the two bones in the forearm that lead to the wrist, the radius and the ulna, are the most likely to fracture. A wrist usually fractures from a fall.

A wrist fracture is often written off as a sprain or a bruise, and you may not see a physician for some time. I have seen many patients complain of a sprained wrist that wouldn't heal and which turned out to be a fracture.

You may also fracture the small bone in the wrist just behind the base of the thumb, called the navicular bone. This fracture is usually caused by stretching your hand out to break a fall.

Even if you do go to a doctor soon after your injury, the navicular fracture may not be apparent on the first X ray because the fracture line is too fine to see. If you feel chronic pain in your wrist that doesn't respond to simple treatments, have it x-rayed once right away and then again 10 days to two weeks later to confirm the diagnosis. By that time, the fracture line will have widened as a result of the healing process.

Healing is more difficult for this fracture than for most other fractures in the body because you may not have an adequate blood supply to the broken bone. It can take eight weeks to eight months for this bone to heal by itself. There are new techniques, however, such as implanting an electromagnet in the cast, that speed bone healing. A magnet works by making the underlying filaments of the bone matrix line up with the same polarity. The filaments tend to get jumbled up at the fracture line, and if you can get them to line up, they form a bridge that can cross the fracture line. A magnet is now commonly used when there is no evidence of healing after a reasonable amount of time, about six weeks.

Finally, if the bone does not reknit, it probably will need to be fixed surgically. You may need a bone graft, which entails taking a piece of bone from the pelvis and placing it across the two bone fragments into a groove. This acts to hold the two pieces together and forms a bridge to help the fracture heal.

If left untreated, the navicular fracture will lead to chronic pain in the wrist and loss of the ability to extend the wrist backward.

MD *Racquet Wrist*

Tennis players also often develop pain at the base of the hand below the pinky finger. Every time the player hits a ball, the racquet butt bangs into and bruises one of the small bones of the wrist. This usually occurs because the racquet butt is too big for the player's hand.

If the pain is severe, you should see a doctor because the little hook of bone at this spot might be broken. If it is, then it will need to be treated as a fracture.

+ *Tendinitis*

The wrist is the passageway for tendons that begin in the forearm and extend into the fingers. The fingers are actually controlled by muscles in the forearm, not in the hand. Overuse of the wrist in sports causes inflammation of the finger tendons attached to these forearm muscles. This results in swelling, pain, and limited function in one or more of the fingers.

Two tendons in the thumb are particularly sensitive to overuse: the extensor and flexor tendons. The extensor tendon moves the thumb away from the second finger, and the flexor tendon moves it toward the second finger. Tendinitis greatly limits your ability to grasp with the thumb. I see many tennis players with pain and swelling on the thumb side of the wrist, which is often caused by gripping the racquet too tightly.

Treatment involves resting and icing the tendon in the wrist, followed by taking anti-inflammatory agents and immobilizing the thumb and wrist to reduce the inflammation.

I normally make a small, lightweight splint for the thumb with pliable plastic that can be removed so that my patient can wash the hand. If the pain is severe, I may also give the patient a cortisone injection.

To prevent the wrist from being overstressed, you need to strengthen the appropriate muscles and tendons. Follow the strengthening exercises outlined in chapter 9. Pay particular attention to Ball Squeezing on page 101. Squeeze to the point of fatigue as many times a day as you can to improve your grip strength.

Finger Flexion and Extension Exercises

You can also improve the extension and lateral movement of your fingers using a rubber band. The large rubber bands used by grocery stores on broccoli or celery provide about the right amount of resistance.

Thumb and Fingers Stretch

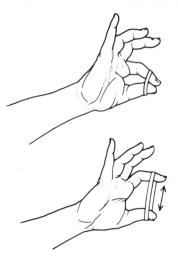

With your palm facing you, hook a rubber band around the thumb and the index finger, and stretch the rubber band between the fingers. Hold for about one second and repeat until fatigued. Then move the rubber band to each of your other fingers and stretch them individually against the thumb.

Thumb and Fingers Flex

To make your fingers stronger in flexion, hook a rubber band around the thumb and one finger, and try to close the finger to the palm. Hold for 5 seconds. Do the same exercise with each of the fingers of the hand.

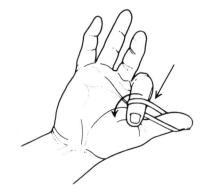

Adjacent Fingers Stretch

Put a rubber band across two adjacent fingers and spread them apart, holding for 5 seconds. Stretch each combination of two adjacent fingers of the hand.

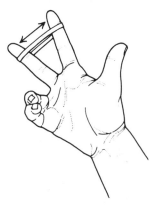

Ganglion

A ganglion is a small lump on the wrist or hand that can vary from the size of a kernel of corn to the size of a cherry. It can occur on the back or front of the wrist, depending if an extensor or flexor tendon is involved. Both of these tendons slide through a sheath lined with cells that produce a slippery, thick fluid. The sheath allows the fingers to make the rapid movements that tennis players depend upon.

If a finger tendon and its sheath become inflamed from overuse or a blow to the wrist, the inflammation can cause part of the tendon sheath to seal off. A cyst forms at this spot because the liquid produced by the sheath is trapped. The cyst, called a ganglion, swells inside the tendon sheath as the cells produce more fluid, and it can become quite painful.

The ganglion may open at one end if there is pressure from overproduction of fluid or from a sudden blow. The increased pressure blows open one end of the cyst, and the fluid runs out. The ganglion then collapses. The problem is that the raw surfaces that have blown out may seal off again, causing the ganglion to reform, and the whole process can repeat itself.

A ganglion becomes a problem when it becomes painful with activity. As long as it doesn't bother you, you don't need to treat it. If pain persists, a doctor can inject the ganglion with cortisone, which causes it to disappear. If the ganglion continues to reform after several injections, then surgical removal may be necessary.

✚ *Carpal Tunnel Syndrome*

The finger tendons pass through the wrist in a narrow, tunnel-like enclosure. With chronic overuse or excessive twisting of the wrist, fluid builds up in the sheath of the tendons, causing the tendons to become inflamed and swollen. Also, the carpal ligament becomes thickened from overuse. Both of these conditions narrow the tunnel and pinch the main nerve that also passes through the tunnel to the fingers.

The result is a painful wrist known as carpal tunnel syndrome, named after the carpal ligament that goes across the top of this tunnel. The pain extends up into the forearm and down into the hand, and may cause numbness, tingling, and even loss of strength in the middle and ring fingers. Anyone who tightly grips something while exercising, such as a tennis racquet, may suffer carpal tunnel syndrome.

The treatment is to rest the affected wrist and apply ice. If the symptoms do not subside, then anti-inflammatory agents may help. Many people will need a splint to minimize or prevent pressure on the nerve and/or a steroid injection into the ligament to help reduce the swelling. If the pain persists, surgery to cut the ligament at the bottom of the wrist may be the only way to release the pressure.

To help you avoid repetitive motion injuries, here are two stretching exercises.

Stretching Exercises

Fingertip Pull

Rest one forearm on a table, and then grasp the fingertips of that hand and pull back gently. Hold for 5 seconds. Repeat with each of the fingers of the other hand.

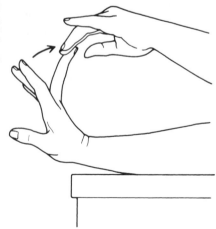

Palm Press

Press your palm flat on a table, as if doing a push-up, and lean forward to stretch the forearm muscles and wrist. Hold for 5 seconds.

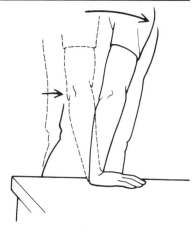

THE HAND

Because the hand is so complex and so vital to everyday activities, all hand injuries should be considered serious and seen by a doctor. You can do irreparable damage by not getting immediate treatment to identify a broken bone. Any rotation of a broken finger bone can compromise that finger's function. Dislocations need to be x-rayed, even if the finger easily pops back into place. A dislocated finger also needs to be immobilized so that the ligaments can heal, or it may dislocate again with much less pressure on the finger.

The locker room saying that "It can't be broken because I can move it" is a myth. All kinds of fractures of the hand allow you to still move the hand. If your hand hurts enough for you to suspect a broken bone, it's best to have it x-rayed.

✚ Abrasions

When reaching for a shot, you may fall on an outstretched hand and suffer abrasions of the palm, or abrasions on the back of your racquet hand or its fingers. On rough playing surfaces, particularly on clay courts, abrasions may occur on any exposed skin surface.

Abrasions should be washed well with soap and water, and an antibiotic ointment applied to them to prevent infection. I prefer to leave the area uncovered unless the abrasions are very unsightly or very painful. If unsightly or painful, they should be covered with a sterile dressing.

Use a nonstick type of pad so that healing tissue is not removed when you change the dressing.

Trigger Finger

Trigger finger is the result of repeated trauma to the palm of the hand. This may be from a tennis racquet jamming into the palm. The trauma causes injury to the flexor tendon to one of the fingers. The tendon's sheath thickens, leaving a narrowed area for the tendon, and the tendon itself also thickens. Consequently, it becomes difficult for the thickened part of the tendon to get through the narrowed part of the sheath.

The flexor muscles of the fingers, which are stronger than the extensor muscles, are strong enough to pull on the tendon and bend the finger. But the extensors are not strong enough to pull it back. The finger ends up in a bent position, the same position of a finger that has pulled the trigger on a gun. The only way to straighten out the finger is to pull on it with the other hand.

This injury sometimes responds to cortisone injection, which reduces inflammation in the tendon sheath. If not, the sheath needs to be split surgically to allow free motion of the finger.

Blisters and Calluses

Many tennis players suffer blisters and calluses on their hands and fingers from gripping the racquet. This often occurs when you switch grips.

Blisters form on the skin when the skin is damaged by friction or burns. Sweat makes your skin sticky, and the friction between your hands and fingers and the racquet can cause blisters.

There are two theories on treating blisters. One says to leave the blisters alone and allow them to heal. New skin forms under the blister and the fluid in it gradually becomes absorbed. Eventually, the outer layer of skin sloughs off.

The other theory suggests opening up the blister and letting the fluid drain out. Then you snip away the dead skin and apply an antibiotic cream to the area and cover it with a Band-Aid or dressing.

I prefer the first method because the second one leaves the raw skin under the blister painful and open to infection. If a blister breaks or becomes damaged by further friction, then use an antibiotic ointment and dressing. If it becomes infected, see a physician.

Calluses are areas of skin that have thickened because of constant pressure. The pressure causes the tissues underneath the callus to become tender. If the callus becomes bothersome, you can soften it with a cream or ointment and rub away dead skin with a pumice stone. If this does not help, a physician can trim the callus surgically or chemically. The great baseball pitcher Nolan Ryan used to soak his hands in pickle brine, which apparently worked for him, though I can't recommend it for everyone.

To prevent these uncomfortable annoyances, you need to find out what is causing them. You may not be holding the racquet properly. Or you may need new grips.

If you sweat a lot, use talcum powder or baby powder during play. Or try using petroleum jelly or tape on problem areas of your grip.

Hand Rehab and Injury Prevention

The rehabilitation of hand injuries is so complex that you should seek out a specialist in hand therapy. Under the specialist's direction, you can usually rehabilitate your hand with exercises at home.

There's not much you can do to prevent hand injuries since most of them are caused by accidents. You can use golf or batting gloves to prevent minor problems, such as blisters and calluses.

If you feel persistent pain in your hand from playing tennis, get your racquet size evaluated immediately. Don't wait because you may have developed a fracture.

Strong fingers are important in almost every sport. They are especially important in tennis so you can hold the racquet lightly but securely. Following is one simple finger-strengthening exercise.

Finger Stretch

Hold your hands out in front of you, palms facing each other and fingers straight up. Bend your fingers down and squeeze them as tightly as you can. Hold for 5 seconds and then release. Repeat five times a day for stronger fingers and a better grip.

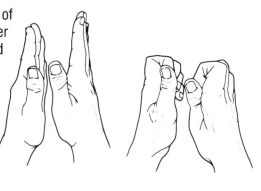

11

The Thigh and Hip

THE THIGH

The thigh contains the major leg muscles. The hamstring muscle in the back of the thigh is the driving force in all running sports, including tennis. Your hamstrings help determine how fast and strong a runner you are. The large quadriceps muscle in the front of the thigh straightens the knee, which helps you stand tall, and is the main muscle used in jumping.

✚ *Hamstring Pull*

The hamstring muscles are often ignored in weight training in deference to their stronger, more aesthetically appealing counterparts, the quadriceps muscles. The hamstrings are implicated in maladies ranging from low-back pain to jumper's knee.

Probably the most common injury in the thigh and hip area, and *the* most common muscle pull, is the hamstring pull. Any rapid running subjects the hamstring muscles to great force; consequently, they are prone to pull. These muscles have an extremely wide range of motion, and stretch out rapidly during the long running stride as you throw your foot forward.

If you pull a hamstring, it may feel as if the muscle has "popped." You will feel a sharp pain and see swelling in the thigh, and maybe even bleeding, depending on the degree of muscle damage. The back of your thigh may turn black and blue, usually right below the area of pain, because blood works its way down by gravity. If you touch the back of the thigh, you may feel a gap in the muscle where the fibers have torn. You will not be able to raise your leg straight off the ground more than 30° to 40° without feeling severe pain.

Rehabilitation begins with the classic use of rest, ice, and compression. The amount of rest depends on the severity of the pull or tear, and is typically two to three days of rest. This should be followed by limited activity until you are free of pain and fully restretched. Icing the muscle for 20 minutes three or four times a day will reduce the chances of aggravating the condition. Then you can start on a gentle stretching program.

You need to start stretching as soon as possible while the muscle is recovering. As long as the stretch is gentle and steady, you can start as early as the second day after your injury, unless you have a major tear. Go into the stretch slowly without jerking the muscle to avoid pulling or tearing it again. Stretch to the point of discomfort, not pain.

The best hamstring stretch is a hurdler stretch. This can be done either sitting (see below) or standing. See the Hurdler Stretch (Standing) on p. 92 in chapter 8.

Hurdler Stretch (Sitting)

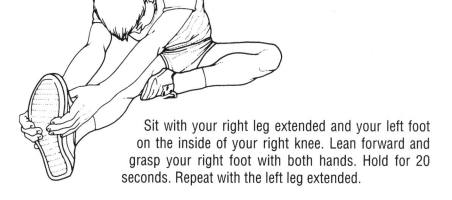

Sit with your right leg extended and your left foot on the inside of your right knee. Lean forward and grasp your right foot with both hands. Hold for 20 seconds. Repeat with the left leg extended.

To prevent another pull or tear, you need to warm up adequately and stretch before playing and, as always, restretch afterward.

Try to keep up your aerobic conditioning and overall muscle tone during your rehabilitation, which may take several months. Cycling and swimming are safe and effective exercises, and should be done pain-free to prevent overstressing the injured muscle.

MD *Sciatica*

The symptoms of sciatica can mimic a hamstring pull with pain in the back of the thigh. I see many patients who complain of a pulled hamstring but who really have sciatica.

Sciatica is simply a symptom or signal that something is irritating the sciatic nerve. Possible causes include a disc in the lower spine pushing on the nerve root where it comes out of the spinal cord; an arthritic spur on the spine pushing on the nerve root; a muscle spasm in the large lower-back muscles, which pulls and stretches the nerve; or a nerve entrapped in the buttock area.

If the thigh pain extends below the knee or if you feel any numbness in your lower leg or foot, the problem is not a hamstring pull but sciatica. If the pain in the back of your leg becomes worse with stretching, then it's probably sciatica and you should see a doctor.

✚ *Quad Pull or Tear*

The large quadriceps muscle is also prone to pulling or tearing during bursts of activity, such as sprinting for a drop shot. However, a quadricep injury poses an additional problem: Blood in the quadriceps will cause calcium deposits to form, a condition called myositis ossificans. If this condition is not treated vigorously, the calcium will not allow the fibers in the muscle to extend fully, which interferes with your speed, and you won't be able to bend your knee all the way. This is a difficult condition to treat and can disable you for up to a year.

A pull or tear to a quadriceps muscle is less common than a hamstring pull or tear. But the treatment is the same—rest the muscle for a few days, then ice and stretch it. You can compress the muscle to prevent bleeding, but do not take anti-inflammatory medications for several days after the injury since anti-inflammatories can increase bleeding. If you have more than mild swelling or pain, see a doctor for a physical therapy prescription.

Prevention is also the same: warm up correctly and stretch the muscle in the front of the thigh through an exercise such as the following.

Quadriceps Stretch

Stand next to a wall and pull the foot of the injured leg towards the buttocks with your hand. Balance yourself against the wall with the other hand. Hold for 15 to 20 seconds and then relax. Repeat five times.

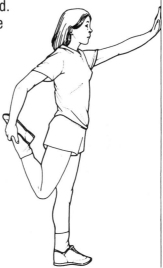

THE HIP

The hip is a very tight, stable, ball-and-socket joint. Because the ball of the hip fits so tightly into the hip socket, it doesn't dislocate like the shallow shoulder joint, and is much less prone to injury. To dislocate a hip, you almost have to be hit by a truck.

EMERGENCY *Broken Hip*

A broken hip causes severe pain and the inability to move the hip or even walk. If you are lying on your back on the court after breaking your hip, your leg may appear to be shortened and your foot rolled to the outside while the other foot points up.

Usually, a broken hip needs to be repaired surgically. This injury is rare among young athletes. It usually occurs in the elderly, who have brittler bones, after suffering a fall.

✚ *Buttock Pull*

A pull of the muscle in the buttock (gluteal muscle) will cause pain there, particularly in response to any physical effort. It will hurt to do a straight leg raise. Doing the Hurdler Stretches will help relieve this minor problem, which should go away within a week or two.

✚ *Groin Pull*

If you make a sudden lateral movement while rotating the leg while running, you can pull a groin muscle. Several different groups of muscles attach to the groin area. The adductor muscles bring one leg in against the other leg, the flexor muscles bend the hip, and the rotator muscles bring the knee across the opposite leg. To determine which muscle is involved, you must find out which motion brings on the pain.

The adductor muscles are pulled when your foot suddenly slides out to the side and overstretches. You feel the pain on the inner part of the thigh. If the injury is not severe, a few days of rest, icing, and taking anti-inflammatories should suffice. Follow this by stretching the muscle with the Groin Stretch (page 11).

In more severe cases, some of the adductor muscle's fibers may tear. You may find a black-and-blue area, which indicates bleeding, that extends from the damaged area down your leg due to gravity. An injury this severe requires rest, stretching, and a strengthening program after the tear has healed.

The hip flexor muscles help throw the leg forward as you walk or run. These muscles can pull or tear as you take off to run forward, such as following your serve to the net. You will feel pain in the front part of the thigh, not the inner surface.

Treatment is the same: rest, ice, and anti-inflammatories, followed by stretching. Do the Hip Extension exercise described on page 94 in chapter 8.

When the rotator muscles pull, you feel the pain in the upper part of the groin area. These muscles pull from twisting or lunging for a ball. If the pull is very mild, use the same treatment described before. But if the pain is moderate to severe, see a doctor because a tear in a rotator muscle can lead to a hernia.

The rotators respond to the Yoga Lotus Stretch.

Yoga Lotus Stretch

While sitting down, bend your knees so that the soles of your feet are touching each other. Now put your elbows on your knees and gradually push them out toward the side. Hold for 20 to 30 seconds.

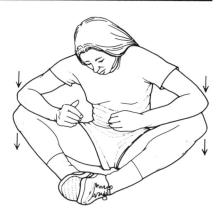

✚ Iliotibial Band Syndrome

The fibrous band running down the outside of the thigh is called the iliotibial band. It provides lateral stability to the hip so that it can't move too far to the outside. In some people, particularly runners, the band overdevelops, tightens, and saws across the hipbone. Each time the runner flexes and bends the knee, the band rubs against bone, causing pain. Although this condition often causes knee pain, it may also cause pain over the point of the hip. (For more about iliotibial band syndrome, see chapter 12.)

A snapping pain in your hip is almost always due to the iliotibial band snapping back and forth over the point of the hip. As you stretch the band out, this pain will disappear.

Knee-over-Leg Stretch (Iliotibial Band Stretch)

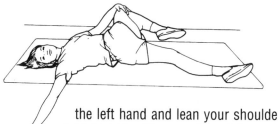

While lying flat on your back, bend your right leg and bring it across your body to the left side. Hold the right knee down with the left hand and lean your shoulders and head back to the right. Hold for 20 seconds and then repeat on the other side.

12

The Knee

The knee is a complex joint that does not simply bend and straighten; it also twists and rotates. The knee depends heavily on the soft tissues that surround it—the muscles, tendons, and ligaments—because it's a weight-bearing joint that is subjected to many different types of motion. This variety of motion can lead to tearing of the cushioning cartilage inside the knee and of the supporting ligaments on both sides of and inside the knee.

Because of its structure, the knee can be severely damaged by rotating, twisting forces. The joint is very well-designed for the functions it was meant to do. But it is the least well-designed of all the joints in the body to withstand the forces of athletics, including tennis. However, modern medicine has responded to the challenge, and even top professionals, including Steffi Graf and Thomas Muster, have returned after devastating knee injuries. And Billie Jean King overcame six knee operations in her career.

✚ SPRAINED KNEE

A knee sprain, by definition, means an injury to a knee ligament. The sprain may vary in severity from a slight stretch to a complete tear of the ligament. A mild, or grade 1, sprain simply stretches the ligament and causes pain and swelling. A moderate, or grade 2, sprain partially tears the ligament and is much more disabling. A severe, or grade 3, sprain is a complete rupture and often needs surgical repair.

The most commonly sprained knee ligament is the medial collateral ligament (MCL). This type of sprain is caused when your foot is planted in the ground. You will feel tenderness and pain on the inside of the knee and feel like the knee will buckle or give way to the inside. Anything more than minimal pain should be treated by a doctor.

The immediate treatment for a sprained knee is the standard RICE formula (see chapter 3). Rest the knee while it aches and ice it intermittently several times a day. Wrap it in an elastic bandage in between ice applications and keep it elevated as much as possible.

If the MCL sprain is mild, an early rehabilitation program using a stationary bicycle and leg extension and curl exercises is all you will need.

Begin by riding a stationary bicycle for 20 minutes. Keep the seat high so that your range of motion is minimal. Don't put any drag on the bike. You are simply interested in moving the knee. In the very beginning, you may not be able to turn the pedal all the way around. Just pedal back and forth until you can come over the top. Once you can do this, start lowering the seat so that you increase the bend in your knee each day until you get back your full range of motion.

Do the Leg Extension exercise while seated at a bench or a table (see page 27 in the strength-training program). Once you lift the weight, hold it at full extension for 3 seconds and then very slowly lower your leg again. Concentrate on the slow movement down. This is the most important part of the lift. Muscle contraction against weight while the muscle is lengthened builds the most muscle strength.

Ten lifts make a set. Do five sets of this exercise. Rest for 30 seconds or more, if needed, after each set. Start with no weight and gradually add weights (5 pounds for men, 2.5 pounds for women) until you have reached the amount of weight necessary for you to fail during the last set. Use ankle weights, a weight boot, or hang an old tote bag or pocketbook filled with weight from the ankle.

Do the Leg Curl while lying on your stomach (see page 28 in the strength-training program). Again, do 10 lifts per set and five sets. If you are using weight machines, hold for 3 seconds with the leg bent. If you are using free weights, this is not necessary.

The purpose of these exercises is to strengthen the quadriceps muscles in the front of the thigh (Leg Extensions) and the hamstring muscles in the back of the thigh (Leg Curls). These muscles, particularly the quadriceps, begin to lose strength within 12 hours of a knee injury. These muscles control the knee and must be restrengthened.

If you have a problem doing the Leg Extensions—that is, if your range of motion is too limited or you find it too painful—then do isometric quadriceps exercises first.

Isometric Quad Exercise

While sitting in a chair, fully extend your leg and tighten your quadriceps muscle to pull the kneecap up. Hold for one second and then relax. Repeat 50 times. The whole exercise should take about 1-1/2 minutes. Do this exercise once an hour while you are awake.

If this exercise is painful with your leg in full extension or if you have trouble controlling the muscle

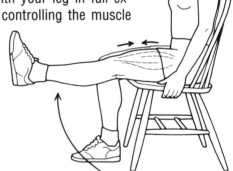

isometrically, you can bend your knee slightly, hook your foot under something too heavy to lift—such as a bed, dresser, or desk—and attempt to lift it. This accomplishes the same thing.

Anything more severe than a minimal knee sprain should be seen by a physician. You will need to begin a rehabilitation program that consists of more sophisticated strengthening exercises, perhaps using isokinetic machines, bracing, and physical therapy.

MD THE CRUCIAL CRUCIATES

If the force to the side of the knee is more severe, or if you are rotating your knee when you are hit by another player, then the anterior cruciate ligament (ACL) may be stretched or torn. Probably the most severe ruptures I see are not caused by trauma but by an athlete running and planting his foot and turning 90°. This is the same motion as planting your foot and rotating sharply to hit the ball.

If your ACL ruptures, the loud pop may be heard by your doubles partner or even your opponents. You will feel sudden pain and instability in the knee. The knee will swell up rapidly because the ACL bleeds quickly when injured. Any ACL injury should cause enough symptoms for you to seek professional help. You cannot self-treat an ACL injury.

A magnetic resonance imaging (MRI) scan may help determine whether the ligament is stretched or totally torn. If it's torn, it will need to be repaired surgically. An older tennis player may be able to get by without surgical repair. Modern methods of repair through the arthroscope plus new ideas on rehabilitation, such as beginning exercises immediately after surgery, have dropped recovery time from 12 to 15 months to 6 to 7 months. Even so, rehabilitation is a major undertaking.

The arthroscope allows complex repairs to be made through a few small holes in the skin. Arthroscopy works best on the knee because the knee has sufficient space for the scope to slip easily around the bones, cartilage, and other tissues. The benefits of successful arthroscopy include less pain, less chance of infection, a shorter recuperation period, and lower medical bills.

There are also rehabilitation programs for partially torn ACLs. Done under a physical therapist's guidance, they center on the use of isokinetic exercise machines, which are much more efficient than regular free weights or the weight machines in gyms. These machines resemble isotonic devices, like the Nautilus leg extension machine, but the isokinetic machines vary the resistance with the amount of pressure applied. The more effort you expend, the more resistance you encounter. Your effort is recorded by a computer and displayed on a screen or printed out on paper.

Once your rehabilitation is complete, very sophisticated knee braces are available that will allow you to return to full activity, even if the ligament has been totally torn and not repaired.

Posterior cruciate ligament (PCL) injuries are very rare. They usually are due to a head-on blow to the knee. You will feel pain and some swelling and cannot accelerate without severe pain. This ligament will usually heal itself.

MD TORN CARTILAGE

A hit on the outer side of the knee causes the inner side to stretch. This can cause two things to happen. The MCL, which is attached to the cartilage, can tear the cartilage as it stretches. Or, when the stretching force is removed, the inner side of the knee closes again with some force, driving the bottom bone of the knee joint back into the cartilage just as a spring hinge of an old screen door slams the door back into the frame.

The grinding action on the knee as it rotates can also damage cartilage. This grinding action is similar to that of a mortar and pestle, with the cartilage the substance being crushed.

If you tear some cartilage, you will feel pain and see swelling in the knee, although not usually as much as with an ACL tear. The pain may be on the inside or the outside of the knee, depending on which cartilage has torn. You may hear a clicking sound inside the knee when you move it. This is the bone riding over the torn part of the cartilage. When you move laterally or twist your knee, the knee may slip and buckle and even cause you to fall. Many of my patients with torn cartilage complain that they can't make a sharp turn even when walking.

The knee may be locked so that it is impossible to extend it fully or bend it. Remember, the knee is a hinged joint, and if a piece of cartilage tears and flops over, it impedes the hinge from working. Just as sticking a pencil in a door will prevent the door from closing all the way, the knee joint won't open or close fully if a piece of cartilage is stuck between the two bones.

Most cartilage tears do not heal by themselves. Cartilage has a poor blood supply except at their outer rim, so about 90 percent of cartilage tears have no ability to heal. Tearing a cartilage is similar to tearing a fingernail. A torn fingernail won't heal by itself; you have to wait for the nail to grow out, and then you cut off the torn part.

Unfortunately, cartilage does not grow back, but the torn piece has to be cut out. The most common way is to shave down the ragged edges of the tear with tiny instruments manipulated through an arthroscope.

Arthroscopic surgery is minor surgery in an expert surgeon's hands. There is no real excuse for opening up a knee for a cartilage repair except in the most unusual cases.

If the tear is at the outer edge of the cartilage, or if it is small, it may heal. Healing requires a rehabilitation program similar to that described for the MCL to restrengthen the muscles around the knee. By following the rehabilitation program, you can usually return to full activity within 3 or 4 weeks.

MD DISLOCATED KNEECAP

The kneecap (patella) is the bone that covers the tendon that runs from the large quadriceps muscle in the front of the thigh to the bone beneath the knee. This tendon is responsible for holding the leg straight so that you can stand erect, and also for straightening a bent leg for climbing stairs and riding a bicycle.

The back of the kneecap is shaped like a wedge and rides in a V-shaped groove in the front of the lower end of the thighbone between the two bottom bones of the knee. If the kneecap is hit at an angle, it can be knocked out of this groove. The kneecap almost always dislocates to the outside since the outer lip of the groove is much shallower than the inner lip.

A dislocated kneecap causes pain, and the knee will appear to be deformed since the kneecap will sit way out to the side. Usually, it can be popped back into place by a doctor without too much difficulty. It may even pop back in by itself on your way to the doctor's office or emergency room. Even if it pops back in, however, you must have it x-rayed to make sure that a piece of bone has not been knocked off the undersurface. Occasionally, the kneecap is locked out of place so severely that surgery is needed to put it back in place.

A dislocated kneecap requires immobilization in a splint for about 3 weeks to allow the tissues on either side of the kneecap to heal. These tissues are responsible for holding it in place, and if they remain torn, the kneecap may be prone to dislocate again. Interestingly, the kneecap groove is much shallower in females than males, so dislocation is a more common, recurring problem among females.

After a period of rest, you must strengthen the quadriceps with a program similar to the one outlined above for the knee ligaments. Start with isometrics and then progress to Leg Extensions (page 27 in chapter 1). These exercises will tighten the kneecap back down by increasing the tone of the muscles pulling on the tendon underneath it. This will hold the kneecap in the groove so that it won't be likely to pop out again.

✚ RUNNER'S KNEE

The most common overuse injury to the knee, and the most common cause of knee pain, is runner's knee or walker's knee, known medically as chondromalacia patella or patello-femoral syndrome. This is due to a misalignment of the kneecap in its groove. The kneecap normally goes up or down in the groove as the knee flexes or straightens. If the kneecap is misaligned, it will pull off to one side and rub on the side of the groove. This causes both the cartilage on the side of the groove and the cartilage on the back of the kneecap to wear out. On occasion, fluid will build up and cause swelling in the knee.

As a result, you will experience pain around the back of the kneecap or in the back of the knee after running. You also will have difficulty going up and down stairs and running hills. It will become painful to sit still for long periods with the knee bent. This is called the "theater sign" of runner's knee because people can't sit through an entire movie or play without getting up to move around. Most likely half of the people you see outside their cars along the roadside are not going to the bathroom; they are stretching their legs to relieve the discomfort of runner's knee.

The basis for the problem is not the knee but the foot. An inward roll of the foot and ankle causes the shinbone to rotate to the inside, which turns the knee to the inside as well. The kneecap ends up sliding at an angle instead of straight up and down.

Treatment involves correcting the foot strike by propping up the foot with an arch or orthotic device inside the tennis shoe. This prevents excessive pronation and keeps the knee in alignment. I suggest you start with just a commercial arch support and progress to a handmade orthotic if you don't get suitable relief.

You also need to do exercises to strengthen the inner side of the quadriceps muscle. The muscle in the front of the thigh hooks into the kneecap and helps align it into the center of the groove. Normally, you strengthen the quadriceps with the full Leg Extension (see page 27). However, in runner's knee, as the quadriceps contracts, it pulls the kneecap back into the groove and grinds it against the side as you lift your calf. So you cannot do the full range of leg extensions with the knee bent without worsening your symptoms.

There is a way to get around this. The inner side of the quadriceps muscle comes into play only in the last 30°, or 6 to 8 inches, as you extend your leg fully. At this point the kneecap is up out of the groove. The idea is to work the quadriceps only within these last 6 to 8 inches of the lift, as described in the 30° Leg Extension.

30° Leg Extension

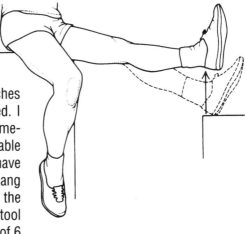

If you are exercising with ankle weights or free weights in a tote bag, put something under your foot so that your heel can come down only 6 to 8 inches after your leg is fully extended. I recommend that you sit on something high, such as a kitchen table or a desk, so that you have enough room for a bag to hang from the ankle without hitting the floor. Then take a chair or stool and pile books on it to a level of 6 to 8 inches below your heel when your leg is fully extended. As you come down, your heel will hit the books and stop your knee from bending.

If you are exercising at home on a bench with a leg machine, put a cinder block or box under the bar so that your leg stops 6 to 8 inches below full extension.

If you are exercising on a weight machine, first stack the weights to full extension. Then have someone else put a second pin into the stack so that when the weights come down 6 to 8 inches, the pin blocks them from going any further.

Do five sets of 10 repetitions with whatever weight it takes until your muscle is exhausted during the fifth set. When the exercise gets easy, move up in weight. Do this once a day every day until you are free of pain. Then do it two or three times a week to keep the quadriceps muscle strong.

If you are doing any other leg-strengthening routines, stay away from leg presses or squats, which put stress on the bent knee. Bending the knee more than 30° will cause symptoms to flare up, so any kind of bent-leg exercise is bad.

The same principle goes for riding a stationary bicycle. The seat should be as high as possible so that you bend your knee as little as possible. Avoid using a StairMaster because climbing steps is particularly worrisome. A stepper on which you can adjust the height of the step is okay if you use a very short step.

A large dose of aspirin also is helpful in stimulating the regeneration of cartilage in the kneecap. Take two plain or buffered aspirin pills with food or milk four times a day until your knee is better. If you have stomach problems, buffered aspirin is better than plain aspirin.

✚ ILIOTIBIAL BAND SYNDROME

Pain along the outer side of the knee is often due to iliotibial band syndrome. The pain usually begins 10 to 20 minutes into your game and gets progressively worse until you are forced to stop. As soon as you stop, the pain almost always goes away. Then it won't bother you until the next time you play. Ten to 15 minutes into your game, it comes back and intensifies the longer you play. If the condition persists, the pain starts earlier and earlier.

The cause of the pain is an overly tight iliotibial band. This is the hard band of fiber you feel in the outside of the thigh extending down to the knee. The band starts at the rim of the pelvis, crosses the point of the hip, comes down the thigh across the outer side of the knee, and attaches below the knee. It helps keep the hip from moving too far to the outside, sort of like the check rein you see on the outside of a racehorse's leg.

Sometimes the band overdevelops and tightens with exercise. When you are running on the court, the band saws against the bony ridge on the outside of the knee as you bend and straighten your leg. It rubs hard enough to irritate the knee, and may also cause similar pain right over the point of the hip.

Treatment is quite easy: All you need to do is stretch the band (see the Knee-over-Leg Stretch on page 121 in chapter 11). You will feel discomfort or pain in the buttock area right behind the bony prominence of the hip due to the band stretching.

Since the band is all in one piece, stretching it in the upper part will loosen it all the way down, and you will no longer feel pressure against the side of the knee. Do three repetitions of this stretch, holding for 20 to 30 seconds. Do this five or six times a day until you can feel the band is loose and no longer causes pain while running. This stretch should become part of your daily routine. If the pain is not better in 10 to 14 days, see a doctor.

13

The Lower Leg

Practically all of the pains that occur on the inner side of the shinbone (tibia) are due to improper foot strike, the way the foot hits the ground when you walk or turn. These are overuse injuries, and the symptoms depend on the amount of stress you place on your legs and the problems you have with your foot strike. A tennis player with a mild foot abnormality may suffer severe shin pain.

Pronation is the inward roll of the foot as it hits the ground. Two different foot problems cause excessive pronation. A person with a pronating foot has an overly mobile foot and ankle and loose ligaments. The foot rolls to the inside when weight is applied to it, as during walking or running. People with pronating feet may say they are flat-footed, and they may be, but often the arch of the foot appears to be rolled down because the ankle collapses inward. The feet and ankles naturally tip inward like those of a beginning ice skater.

The other problem is Morton's foot, which is characterized by the second toe being longer than the big toe. If you have Morton's foot, your foot will roll to the inside when you come up on your toes to push off for the next step. (See chapter 15 for more about specific foot problems.)

Excessive pronation can lead to three lower leg injuries: shinsplints, tibial stress syndrome, and tibial stress fractures.

✚ SHINSPLINTS

"Shinsplint" is a wastebasket term used for any pain on the inner side of the shin. A true shinsplint is quite rare.

What people call shinsplints are actually pains in the muscles near the shinbone. They can be caused by running or jumping on hard surfaces. They usually occur in people unaccustomed to training, although they can also plague experienced athletes who switch to lighter shoes, harder surfaces, or more concentrated speed work.

The pain is felt on the inner side of the middle third of the shinbone, which is where the muscle responsible for raising the arch of the foot attaches. When the arch collapses with each foot strike, it pulls on the tendon that comes from this muscle.

The arch collapses to absorb the shock of the foot hitting the ground. As you come up on your toes for the next stride, the muscle attached to the arch fires and pulls the arch back up to ready it for the next impact. This muscle responds totally to the stretch of the tendon as the arch flattens.

In people who excessively roll their ankles to the inside (pronate), the arch stays down. Consequently, the muscle starts to fire while there is still weight on the foot, and it is unable to bring the arch up. Because of its multiple firings during each foot strike and its pull against great weight, the arch muscle tears some of its fibers loose from the shinbone. This causes small areas of bleeding around the lining of the bone and pain.

Much more common among tennis players is the bone stress syndrome. When the ankle rolls over, it rotates the shinbone to the inside with each step while the upper part of the leg remains almost fixed. This abnormal twisting of the bone, coupled with the fact that you come down with two to four times your body weight on your leg when you run, puts stress on the shinbone and causes irritation and pain.

The key element in treatment is an arch support to prevent excessive pronation and pull on the tendon. For beginning pain, propping up the foot with an arch support usually solves the problem almost immediately. For bone stress, it may take 2 to 3 weeks to become pain-free. Most tennis players do well with a simple commercial arch support. If you have a more serious problem, you may need an orthotic device custom-made by a sports podiatrist. Icing the sore shin and taking anti-inflammatory medications may also help ease the pain. As soon as the rotation stops, the soreness will begin to disappear, and you should be pain-free in two to three weeks.

🄼🄳 STRESS FRACTURE

If the twisting of the shinbone is severe and prolonged enough, the bone may become fatigued and crack, just as a piece of metal may do. This is called a stress fracture, and is the last and most disabling of these shin injuries. A stress fracture will need 6 to 8 weeks of rest.

Your body can compensate for this stress to some extent. X-ray studies of the shinbone show that the bone thickens in an attempt to strengthen itself. But if you continue to play and the bone fails to strengthen itself sufficiently, it can develop a minute, often microscopic, crack, or stress fracture.

The problem with identifying a stress fracture is that the crack is so small that it typically cannot be seen on an X ray until it begins to heal itself a few weeks later. If your leg X ray is negative and you still feel shin pain, then you should have a bone scan. This is a simple, safe X ray procedure that will reveal a stress fracture within 24 to 48 hours of the injury.

You should suspect a stress fracture if the pain level of bone stress syndrome suddenly increases. Also, if you previously felt pain only while running and you now feel it while walking, you may have a stress fracture.

A tibial stress fracture requires rest. You cannot play through it; it will only get worse, and the crack in the bone will get larger. If the pain becomes severe, you may need crutches to walk. Otherwise, a break from playing for 6 to 8 weeks should be enough. You can cycle or swim for exercise, if this causes you no pain.

As the fracture heals, treat it with one of the support devices mentioned earlier. If you don't correct your foot strike, you will likely fracture the bone again.

✚ PAIN ON THE OUTSIDE OF THE LEG

Another type of pain occurs on the outer part of the lower leg and is due to stress on the small bone on the outside of the leg (fibula). This, however, is due to pounding and shock transmission up the outside of the leg rather than twisting.

This type of pain occurs mostly among people with a supinating foot—one that rolls to the outside because the arch is too tight. This is a high-arched, rigid foot that will not collapse on impact. Look at your shoes and see if they are badly turned over on the outside of your foot when you run. Since the arch of a supinated foot does not collapse to sustain the shock of the foot strike, the shock is transmitted up the outside of the lower leg and can result in bone pain and a possible stress fracture of the fibula.

Treating this condition is much more difficult. You can prop up a loose arch, but you cannot make a tight arch collapse. The best treatment is to provide maximum padding for shock absorption at the outer side of the foot. An air-sole shoe or a very soft-sole shoe is not the answer because the outside of the sole soon collapses, increasing supination. If the padding is not effective, you may need an orthotic device to protect the foot.

Fibula pain is less debilitating because the fibula is not a true weight-bearing bone. The pain should disappear in 2 to 3 weeks with proper padding under the foot.

✚ LEG MUSCLE PULLS AND TEARS

Muscle pulls and tears commonly occur in the major muscles of the calf, the gastrocnemius and the soleus. These muscles make up the large bulge in the back of the lower leg and are responsible for lifting the heel and driving you forward as you run.

Pulls and tears represent different degrees of the same injury as muscles are suddenly overstretched beyond their limits. The degree of overstretching determines whether the muscle is pulled or actually torn.

Treatment depends on the severity of the injury. You should rest for a few days to begin with and then begin a gentle, gradual stretching program. Calf stretches are best done with the Wall Push-up (see page 13). Do the Wall Push-up one leg at a time. If you stretch both legs at the same time and one calf is tighter than the other, which is likely if you have a pulled muscle, you are limiting the stretch of the good leg to what you can do with the bad leg.

As always, adequately stretching the muscle is also the best way to prevent a pull or tear.

Once the muscle is adequately restretched, it should be restrengthened. Toe Raises are the easiest way to do this.

Toe Raise

Stand on your toes for 10 seconds and then come down flat on the floor. Repeat until you feel real fatigue in your calf muscles.

As the calf muscles begin to strengthen, you can put all of your weight on the affected leg and keep the other leg off the floor. Then you can hold dumbbells or a barbell to increase your body weight. Use the unaffected leg for balance, but do all of the lifting with the affected calf.

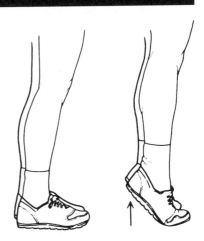

✚ CALF CRAMPS

Calf cramps are dangerous because the sudden muscle pain can be so severe that a runner falls and risks other injury. No one has pinpointed the exact cause of muscle cramps. A number of factors may be at work, including dehydration, electrolyte imbalance in the blood, poor physical conditioning, and improper diet.

A new explanation for cramping points the finger at muscle fatigue, which may cause the nervous system to signal certain muscles to contract. While fatigue doesn't discriminate between those in shape and those who aren't, lack of conditioning does. The fitter your body, the better it transports nutrients like oxygen and glucose to the muscles for fuel. If adequate energy isn't available, the muscle proteins bind to each other and the muscle stays contracted in a cramp.

Calf cramps usually occur after periods of repeated heavy exercise. I see plenty of muscle cramps among tennis players. Some of them sweat profusely or are on low-salt diets, and the cramping may be related to these factors. I tell these tennis players to drink more water before, during, and after practice sessions, and this generally limits the cramping.

Many people assume that a nutritional deficiency is the main cause of muscle cramps, but that's not the case. Over-exercise, fatigue, poor conditioning, and water loss should first be eliminated as causes before you check for any nutritional deficiencies.

The calf muscle often twitches uncontrollably, which is a signal that it may go into spasm. When the muscle does cramp, stretch it out gently by doing Wall Push-ups (see page 13). Then massage the muscle with your thumbs and forefingers from the top down toward your feet until the pain passes.

Playing through a cramp can actually damage muscle fibers and put you out of commission for a few days. When a cramp strikes, stop what you are doing, slowly stretch the muscle, and breathe deeply to help the nervous system release its grip.

✚ ACHILLES TENDINITIS

The Achilles tendon, the largest tendon in the body, is found below the calf and helps lift the heel. It may become inflamed and cause tendinitis, which is a prime symptom of an overuse injury. The most common cause is excessive pronation of the ankle and foot, which cause the Achilles tendon to pull off-center. This condition may also be due to over-stress from frequent jumping.

The treatment for Achilles tendinitis is to rest until it feels better and to ice the tendon several times a day during this time. You can use anti-inflammatory agents to relieve swelling and pain. Stretch the tendon as well with Wall Push-ups or Heel Drops (see page 13).

An arch support or orthotic device may help correct the pronation that caused the tendinitis. Whether you need an arch support or an orthotic depends on the severity or complexity of your foot disability, not on the severity of your tendinitis. A severely pronating foot with lax ligaments will probably respond well to an arch support. A foot that pronates less but has a variety of other problems may not benefit as much from a simple arch. I suggest that every tennis player try an arch first and, if that doesn't work, then go on to an orthotic.

MD ACHILLES TENDON RUPTURE

After enjoying Easter brunch at their tennis club with their best friends, Rick and Andrea, Jodi and her husband, Mark, played a set. "He was beating the pants off me. I just couldn't get into my game," says Jodi, who has been playing tennis all of her life. So frustrated that Mark, a beginning-intermediate player, had beaten her, Jodi insisted that Rick play her a set. "I was so frustrated that my husband had won, I played very aggressively, and ended up putting Rick in the hospital," Jodi says. Rick, who had just gotten off crutches from a major auto accident, ran down one of Jodi's volleys and tore his Achilles tendon. "On the way to the hospital, Rick forgave me, but Andrea had some choice words for me," says Jodi.

The classic case of a ruptured Achilles tendon is a person stepping or lunging and then feeling a snap at the back of the calf. Tennis players often report that it felt as if someone hit them in the back of the heel with the ball. The snap of the tendon may sound like a bone breaking.

A complete tear of the Achilles tendon is thought to be due to an accumulation of frequent, small tears or inflammations that have weakened the tendon. Scar tissue may build up around the tendon, and swelling may be apparent above the heel. Once a rupture occurs, you can often feel a hole between the tendon's severed ends.

One sign of Achilles rupture is the inability to stand on your toes. However, this test is not completely reliable. Also, when you walk, your foot may turn out to the side. A ruptured Achilles tendon can be confused with a partial rupture because it may cause little pain at first. In fact, an Achilles rupture is quite often misdiagnosed. The only foolproof way to know if you have ruptured this tendon is to lie on your stomach with your foot off the end of a bed, toes pointing down, and have someone squeeze your calf. The front of the foot normally will move down. If there is no flex in the foot, then the tendon is torn. You can also compare the two legs. Squeeze the uninjured leg first to observe the flexing movement, and then squeeze the injured leg to see whether it moves.

For a tennis player, the best treatment for this condition is surgical repair. There is a method used for the elderly in which the tendon is placed in a cast, but this is not usually adequate for a tennis player. Ideally, you should have the operation within 2 weeks of the injury. You will be in a cast for 6 to 8 weeks. For the first few weeks the cast will extend above the knee, and then it will be reduced to below the knee.

After 8 weeks you can start range-of-motion and stretching exercises. These will be difficult and should always be done with a physical therapist. It may be 6 months or more until you can return to playing tennis. Coming back from a ruptured Achilles tendon is one of the most difficult recoveries for a tennis player.

🆛 TENNIS LEG

A small tendon, the popliteus tendon, runs parallel to the Achilles tendon on the inside of the leg. It probably no longer has any function, and there is some argument over whether everyone has this tendon. But if you have it and you overstress it suddenly, it can snap.

A popliteus rupture is so common among tennis players, usually as you make the first hard step toward the net, that it is called "tennis leg." It is also referred to as a disease of the aging athlete because it becomes more common with advancing age. Young athletes almost never rupture the popliteus tendon.

The symptoms of a popliteus rupture are similar to those of an Achilles rupture. The victim may complain of being hit in the back of the calf with a tennis ball or a small stone from another court. You also may not be able to stand on your toes and may have a similar gait as someone with an Achilles tendon rupture. The base of the bulging muscle on the inner side of the calf will be quite tender, and you may see a black-and-blue spot there. You will also feel pain if you press on this area.

The treatment is to ice the calf intermittently for the first few days and to rest it. You may need to walk with a cane or crutches during this time. An elastic bandage wrapped around the area and anti-inflammatory medications may also help ease the calf pain. As soon as you can tolerate it, start a gentle stretching program, including Wall Push-ups and Heel Drops (see page 13). As the pain diminishes, you can increase your intensity until you attain full flexibility.

Normally, the symptoms subside in about 2 weeks, and you can return to playing tennis. Don't go back onto the court unless you can stretch the affected side without pain as far as you can stretch the good side. If you go back too soon, you are likely to rupture the tendon again.

As usual, the best prevention is to warm up and stretch properly. This injury is most prevalent among tennis players probably because they are notoriously bad at stretching. This injury should be examined by a physician to differentiate it from an Achilles rupture.

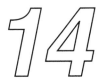

The Ankle

The ankle's structure allows you to move your foot in many directions. The foot's up-and-down movement enables you to walk by first striking the ground with the heel and then pushing off from your toes. Without this movement, you would be able to walk with your foot flat on the floor.

The other important ankle movements are rolling the foot to the inside and to the outside. This allows you to adjust your foot to uneven surfaces so that you can walk on the side of a hill or step on a pebble and not fall.

And there's the rub. When the foot rolls to the outside on an uneven surface, it may continue to roll over until it has stretched and sprained the not-so-strong ligaments on the outside of the ankle. The presence of small holes in playing fields leads to many sprains. Even on a flat surface such as a tennis court, a player can always step on his or her doubles partner's foot and turn the ankle over.

In the ankle, three bones form what is called a mortise joint. The dome of the ankle bone (talus) sits in a squared-off socket formed by the two bones of the lower leg (tibia and fibula). The joint is held together by three moderately strong ligaments on the outside of the ankle and one very large, very strong ligament on the inside.

✚ ANKLE SPRAINS

There are three grades of ankle sprain. When you step gently up onto the court and twist your ankle, you simply stretch the ligaments, with no real tearing. That's a mild, or grade 1, sprain. When you lunge out over a poorly planted foot, partially tearing the fibers of the ligament, that's a moderate, or grade 2, sprain. When you jump and land on your partner's foot, twisting and forcing the ankle violently to the court, most or all of the fibers tear. That's a severe, or grade 3, sprain. A moderate sprain requires vigorous treatment and a severe sprain may put you in a cast or require surgery.

Treat a sprained ankle right, and you can be on your feet in a few days and back in action in a few weeks. A severe or mistreated sprain, however, may not heal for 6 months or more. Therefore, all but the mildest sprains should be medically checked.

An ankle sprain is a fairly common tennis injury, and is more common on hard courts than on Har-Tru or grass.

THE STEPS TO RECOVERY

The best treatment is the RICE formula: rest, ice, compression, and elevation. Your goal is to limit internal bleeding and swelling. If the sprain is severe, you may need to splint the ankle.

Rest your ankle immediately. A sprain's intense pain eases after a few minutes, and you may be tempted to keep playing. But hours later, you may have a sore, swollen, discolored ankle. If you stay off the ankle until the swelling stabilizes, you can usually walk easily within 24 hours. You may need crutches for a day or two.

Ice the ankle until the swelling disappears. The ice curtails bleeding by narrowing blood vessels and helps reduce swelling. Fill a plastic bag with crushed ice and strap it onto the ankle with a towel or elastic bandage. Or you can use a bag of frozen peas or carrots from the supermarket.

Continue icing the ankle for 20 minutes or until it starts to feel numb, and then take off the ice pack and give the ankle enough time to regain some warmth, usually about 20 minutes. Keep icing for 20 minutes on and 20 minutes off for 48 hours or until the ankle returns to normal size.

Compress the ankle in between icings and at night by wrapping it with an elastic bandage, which limits the swelling and bruising.

Elevate the ankle so that it's above your hips and, if possible, above your heart. At night, rest it on pillows or put a suitcase under the mattress at the foot of the bed.

Range-of-Motion Exercises

As soon as you can, begin range-of-motion exercises. These can help reduce stiffness and restore mobility.

Alphabet Range-of-Motion Exercise

Sit in a chair and cross the affected leg over the other leg at the knee. Now, using your big toe as a pointer, trace the capital letters of the alphabet from A to Z. Hold the big toe rigid so all the motion comes from the ankle. Repeat this exercise every hour while you are awake. The letters will be very small at first, but they will increase in size as your range of motion improves.

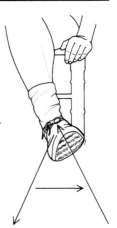

You should try to put weight on the ankle as soon as possible, depending on the severity of the sprain. If you need crutches, put a little weight on your ankle as you use them. You can begin to walk as soon as it feels comfortable. Do not put your full weight on the ankle until you can walk with a normal heel-to-toe gait. Do not duckwalk by turning your foot to the side in order to be rid of the crutches.

Ankle-Strengthening Exercises

Once your range of motion is near normal, you can begin strengthening exercises.

Ankle Lift

Take a piece of rope about 1.5 feet long, and either tie a 5-pound weight to each end or loop the rope around a 10-pound weight. Sit on a counter and drop the rope over the top of the toes (while wearing an athletic shoe). Lift the weight with your ankle as many times as you can.

Ankle Turn

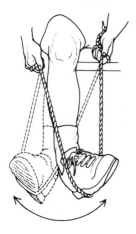

While sitting on a counter, take a long rope, put it under the arch of the shoe of the affected foot, and hold the ends of the rope at about knee height. Turn your ankle as far as it will go to the inside. Now pull on the inside part of the rope and force your ankle to the outside, working against the resistance of the rope. When your foot is all the way out, pull on the outside part of the rope as you bring your foot back to the inside, again working against resistance. Keep the inward and outward movements going until your ankle is fatigued.

Foot Lift (Outward)

While sitting on a counter, hang a weight on your toes, point your foot up, and turn your ankle as far as it will go to the outside. Repeat as many times as you can. Start with a 5-pound weight and work your way up to heavier weights.

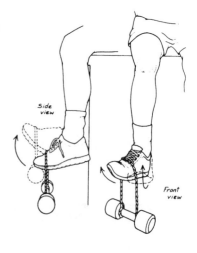

Side view

Front view

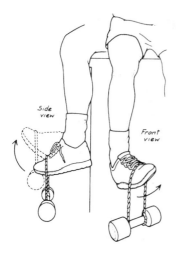

Side view

Front view

Foot Lift (Inward)

While sitting on a counter, hang a weight on your toes, point your foot up, and turn your ankle as far as it will go toward the inside. Repeat as many times as you can. Start with a 5-pound weight and work your way up to heavier weights.

Also do the Toe Raise (see page 135) and Heel Drop (see page 13), alternating them until your ankle is fatigued. As your ankle gets stronger, lift up your good foot and put all your weight on the injured ankle.

Each of these exercises should be done to the point of total muscle fatigue, so that you can't do even one more.

Balancing is important in retraining an injured ankle to sense where the foot is in relation to the ground. Practice by balancing on one foot with your arms stretched out to the sides until you lose balance or become fatigued. When your ankle gets better, do this exercise with your eyes closed.

If the sprain is severe or if you need to make a quick return to playing for a big tournament, you should consider a good physical therapy program. All of the preceding exercises can be done on machines, which are much more effective than weights and pieces of rope. For balance training you can stand on a balancing, or wobble, board, which is a board that rests on a cylinder and allows you to roll back and forth. Balancing on one foot on the board can enhance your ankle stability. These exercises can be combined with electrotherapy, range-of-motion exercises, and massage under the direction of a physical therapist, who knows when and how hard to push you.

PREVENTING ANOTHER ANKLE SPRAIN

The tried-and-true method of protecting a sprained ankle is to wrap the ankle tightly in athletic tape. But that requires learning the intricacies of proper ankle taping. What's more, tape tends to loosen while you play. As an alternative, use a lace-up cloth brace, which can be tightened during a service break. Elastic braces or bandages are of little value in preventing reinjury because they stretch if the ankle starts to turn over again.

If your ankle is still weak, you can use an Air-Cast, which consists of two sets of inflatable bladders that are laced together and run up both sides of the ankle. This brace holds the ankle firm and allows you to run. You can wear it until your ankle is fully restrengthened.

If you have problems with recurring sprains, an orthotic device with a lateral flange or built-up area over the side of the heel can prevent the ankle from turning over. Persistent sprains may require surgical repair of the ankle ligaments.

People with tight ligaments, such as those with a supinating foot or Morton's foot, may have continuing problems. The supinating foot tends to land on the outside and predisposes the ankle to turn out over the foot. Similarly, the tennis player with Morton's foot is susceptible to ankle sprains because the foot lands on the outside, which makes the ankle prone to turn outward.

Ankle sprains should be taken seriously. Follow an aggressive rehabilitation program to speed recovery and reduce the chances of reinjury. Push yourself just to the point of pain; otherwise, rehabilitation may be too conservative and keep you out of action longer than necessary. Maintain your cardiovascular fitness through cycling and walking in water with a flotation belt while you rehabilitate your ankle.

MD *Broken Ankle*

In rare instances, a tennis player can break an ankle if it is turned severely with great force. It's very difficult to differentiate a sprained ankle from a broken one. A large, swollen ankle may only be sprained, whereas a healthier-looking ankle may be broken. For this reason, I recommend that every ankle injury, except the most minimal sprains, be x-rayed.

If a tennis player goes down with a severe ankle injury, the ankle should be splinted and the player sent to an emergency room. It may look silly, but nobody will laugh at a sprained ankle with a splint on it, and splinting will help protect the ankle if it's broken.

Common signs of a difficult-to-spot broken ankle include a recurrent, diffuse ache in the ankle that increases with playing; swelling after playing, followed by pain-free periods; limited movement; bruising in the ankle; and an unremitting ache.

All ankle fractures require medical care and prolonged casting. Suffice it to say that if you break your ankle, you need to see a doctor.

You must also bring the ankle back up to 100 percent strength with a rehabilitation program in order to compete at your previous level without the threat of reinjury.

15

The Foot

The foot is the most complex structure in the lower body. It is made up of many bones that interact, unlike the rest of the structures of the lower body, in which only two or three bones interact.

The main function of the foot is to absorb the shock of the body's weight landing on it. The foot supports up to four times your body weight when you are running fast. It also must lock itself into a rigid position when you come up on your toes to push off so that it can act as a lever of propulsion. And the foot must roll from the outside to the inside as your body weight comes forward from the heel to the front of the foot.

✚ FOOT ABNORMALITIES

Structural abnormalities of the foot can cause stress all the way up the leg into the back. The foot may roll to the inside (pronation) or the outside (supination), or the second toe may be longer than the big toe. These problems can be corrected by commercial arch supports, or if foot pain is persistent, orthotic devices that fit inside the tennis shoe.

Common Types of Foot Abnormalities

Pronating Foot

The pronating foot has loose ligaments and, because it doesn't have the proper support, rolls to the inside. The foot appears to be flat because the arch becomes compressed when the foot rolls over. But when the weight is taken off the foot, the arch reappears. Someone with true flat-feet has no arch at all.

The inward roll of the foot causes the entire leg to rotate to the inside. The kneecaps point toward each other. Everything in the tennis player's leg and hip is pulled out of line. The pronating foot causes any number of conditions up the leg, from heel pain and Achilles tendinitis to shin-splints, bone stress syndrome, and a stress fracture on the inside of the shinbone to disabling kneecap pain.

A pronating foot can be propped up with an arch support under the inside of the foot. This keeps the foot in line when it strikes the ground and prevents the leg from rolling inward.

Supinating Foot

The supinating, or cavus, foot is the mirror image of the pronating foot. The ligaments are tight, and the foot is rigid with a high arch, which causes the tennis player to walk on the far outer portion of the foot. Because the arch is too tight, it cannot collapse when the foot hits the ground. With no arch to absorb the shock of each step, the shock is sent straight up the outside of the leg.

The shock transmission leads to pain on the outer side of the leg. It can cause bone stress syndrome or a stress fracture in the fibula, the small bone on the outside of the shinbone, pain in the outer side of the knee, and even pain extending up into the outer part of the hip.

The supinating foot requires soft padding under the outside of the foot. If you have this problem, I suggest gluing a quarter inch of soft foam padding from a Dr. Scholl's Flexo Arch along the outside edge of the arch of your tennis shoe. This will cause your foot to roll back slightly toward the middle and will provide some padding to reduce the pounding on your leg. Or you may need an orthotic device to take some of the weight off the outer side of the foot.

Morton's Foot

Morton's foot is characterized by the second toe being longer than the big toe. The problem is that the bone behind the big toe (first metatarsal) is too short. This inherited trait occurs in about 25 percent of the population and causes problems in more people than the other two foot abnormalities combined.

When you walk, you create forward momentum by pushing off with the big toe, which is called toeing off. Just before toeing off, you place all of your weight on the head of the first metatarsal. In a tennis player with Morton's foot, the first metatarsal is too short to provide the leverage needed to shift the weight to the bottom of the big toe. Instead, the foot buckles to the inside, and the weight rolls along the inner side of the big toe. This is similar to what happens with the pronating foot, but a Morton's foot doesn't pronate until weight is placed on the toes.

Tennis players with Morton's foot first strike the ground with the far outer part of the foot. This is probably an unconscious attempt to correct the inward roll of the foot, but it doesn't help prevent the pronation on toeing off. Instead, the tennis player ends up walking across the foot, landing on the outside of the heel, and then toeing off on the inside of the big toe, instead of walking with a straight-footed, heel-to-toe gait.

Walking on the inner side of the big toe of a Morton's foot usually forms a large callus there. The big toe will also be pushed toward the second toe, and the pressure on the inside of the big toe may cause bunions on the inside of the foot.

Because the Morton's foot starts on the outside of the foot and then pronates at toe-off, it combines the worst features of both the pronating and supinating foot, and can cause all of the conditions they cause.

If you have Morton's foot, you may get by with a commercial arch support along with a foam pad under the big toe. More likely, you will need an orthotic device that has an arch support and is built up under the big toe joint. When your foot starts to buckle, the built-up area in the orthotic will force you to push straight off your foot.

Telltale Signs of Foot Abnormalities

One of the best ways to diagnose foot problems is to look at the wear patterns in a pair of tennis shoes. A pronating foot wears out the inside of the heel and toe, and the shoe breaks over to the inside. If the shoe is placed flat on a tabletop, it will lean to the inside, particularly the heel counter. A supinating foot wears out the outside of the shoe, from the heel all the way down to the toes. This shoe will lean to the outside. A Morton's foot wears out the shoe on the outside of the heel and at the midsole, and then straight across the sole to the inside of the big toe (see the figure below).

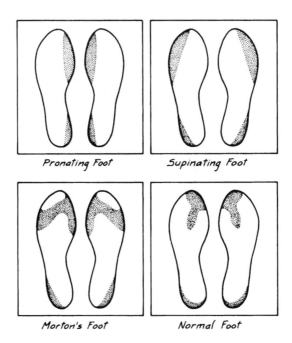

Pronating Foot   Supinating Foot

Morton's Foot   Normal Foot

Orthotics

Orthopedists have begun to question the safety, expense, and usefulness of the rigid, custom-made inserts that have become trendy among tennis players. Orthotic devices contain carefully placed divots and bumps designed to shift your weight in a way that forces you to walk or run more naturally. They are made from a variety of materials, from layered foam to leather-covered cork to hard plastic.

Orthotics are not the answer to all foot problems. In fact, about 80 percent of the tennis players who spend hundreds of dollars for custom-made devices would do just as well with a soft arch support. Many commercial arch supports are available for $15 to $40 at drugstores or sporting goods stores.

I usually don't send a tennis player to be fitted for an orthotic until he or she has failed to improve with a stock arch support. If the foot problem is so complex that a simple stock arch will be ineffective, then I order an orthotic right away.

If you have persistent foot pain that you can't trace to an episode of trauma, put some type of arch in your tennis shoe. If nothing changes, then your pain is not due to an overuse injury, and you need to see a doctor to find out what's wrong. If the pain diminishes or even gets worse, then you probably have an overuse injury. Any change in pain is a sign that the arch support has had some effect. If the pain goes away, continue using the arch support. If the pain gets worse, see a sports podiatrist for a properly fitting orthotic.

In looking for a podiatrist to make an orthotic, it's important to find someone who deals with athletes. A tennis orthotic is very different from a walking orthotic. If you choose someone who doesn't understand the mechanics and stresses of playing tennis, you may end up spending a lot of money for little or no pain relief. Also, wearing an orthotic insert should never be painful. If it is, take it back and have it adjusted.

✚ FOOT PAIN

Pain in the front of the foot just behind the toes (metatarsalgia) can be due to the stress of placing weight on the toes when you play. Usually, you will feel the pain in your second or third toe. The heads of the metatarsal bones in these toes may drop slightly, and the excessive weight placed on them as you come up on your toes causes pain. A pad behind the heads of these toes will lift them and take the weight off, and this usually relieves the pain.

✚ BRUISED FOOT

A tennis player whose foot is stepped on can develop a nasty-looking bruise. If you bruise your foot, ice it for 4 or 5 days and rest it until you can walk normally.

✚ BLACK TOENAILS

I occasionally see tennis players whose toenails turn black and fall off. This is due to the toenail banging into the toe box of the tennis shoe. The constant banging causes bleeding under the toenail, which makes it turn black.

The problem is an undersized shoe. As you play, your foot spreads out and swells up slightly, so your tennis shoes should be one size larger than your dress shoes. Sizes vary from brand to brand, so always try on a new shoe carefully. Regardless of the shoe's stated size, if your toenail turns black after playing, the shoe is too small.

Tennis players with Morton's foot have an additional problem. The toe boxes of tennis shoes are all designed with the assumption that the big toe is the largest toe. In the player with Morton's foot, the second toe is the largest, so most tennis shoes do not fit properly. If you have Morton's foot, try on a lot of styles and see which one is the most comfortable.

✚ PLANTAR FASCIITIS

Pain in the arch or under the heel that occurs while you are walking is called plantar fasciitis. The plantar fascia is the elastic covering that runs the length of the foot, from just behind the toe bones to the heel bone, and holds up the arch. Overstretching this shock-absorbing layer causes pain and inflammation along the length of the arch.

This injury usually happens to tennis players with high, rigid arches. You will feel the pain when pushing off for the next stride or putting weight on the foot. When the arch starts to come down, it stretches the plantar fascia and pulls on its fibers. The torn fibers may go into spasm and shrink. With every step, the plantar fascia tears a little more and causes pain.

The dull pain is particularly bad the first few minutes after rising in the morning or after sitting for a long time. With the weight off your feet, the plantar fascia will start to heal. But each time you again put weight on your foot, the torn fibers will be pulled apart as the arch collapses.

Treatment consists of immediately supporting the arch with a commercial arch support. This will prevent the arch from collapsing and the plantar fascia from stretching. Put an arch support in your slippers and wear them as soon as you get out of bed. Even a few steps without support can stretch the plantar fascia. By using arch supports, you will likely feel relief within 2 to 3 days.

Three out of four tennis players will do well with an inexpensive commercial arch support, while those with a high, rigid arch may need an orthotic for more support.

Plantar fasciitis is particularly common among middle-aged people who have been sedentary and who suddenly increase their level of physical activity. People who begin to play tennis or those who suddenly have time to play more are particularly prone to this condition.

✚ HEEL BURSITIS

Pain in back of the heel where the Achilles tendon attaches to the heel bone can be due to bursitis. Under the Achilles tendon is a small bursal sac, about the size of a bean, that protects the tendon from rubbing on the heel bone. When the Achilles tendon goes out of alignment, a situation usually due to pronation, it puts undue stress on the bursa, and the sac becomes inflamed and painful.

This form of bursitis sometimes responds to an arch support, which brings the Achilles tendon back into alignment. More often, however, it requires a small injection of cortisone, like any other bursitis.

✚ MORTON'S NEUROMA

Pain, numbness, and sensitivity between the third and fourth toes is known as Morton's neuroma. You may also feel the pain between the second and third toes. Squeezing the forefoot can reproduce the pain, which is caused by pressure on the nerves of the toe bones.

A wider tennis shoe may provide relief by easing the pressure. If that does not work, try an orthotic for pressure relief. If that fails, then cortisone injections or surgery may be necessary.

✚ PUMP BUMP

An abnormal, knoblike growth on the back of the heel can be caused by friction and the pressure of the tennis shoe's heel counter on the heel bone. As the weight shifts as you swing, the pressure on the heel bone increases. Not only is this painful, but the Achilles tendon can become inflamed, or the tennis player can develop bursitis at that spot.

The treatment includes a heel cup, which holds and cushions the heel within the shoe; padding; a heel counter, to provide cushioning and support; icing the heel bone intermittently; and anti-inflammatory agents for the bursitis pain. Stretching with the Wall Push-up (page 13) and the Heel Drop (page 13) helps relieve the Achilles tendinitis.

✚ STRESS FRACTURE OF THE FOOT

If you have felt mild pain in your foot for days or even weeks while playing tennis, and you then feel a sudden, severe pain in the front part of your foot while playing, you probably have a stress fracture of the foot. Stress fractures occur most often when you change your workout—for example, by increasing your playing time or switching to hard courts after playing on clay or grass.

When excessive force is transmitted to the second, third, or fourth metatarsal bone, the bone can crack from overfatigue. When you come up to toe off, most of your weight is on the first metatarsal, behind the big toe. This bone is very thick and heavy to provide support. If the bone is too short, as in Morton's foot, your weight will be transmitted to the other toe bones, which are not as heavy. As a result, they can crack.

If you suffer a stress fracture, both the upper and the lower surfaces of your foot will be tender, and you may have some swelling. You will need to get an X ray of the foot, and sometimes even a bone scan, to confirm the diagnosis.

A stress fracture needs rest for 4 to 6 weeks to allow the fracture to heal. Crutches are necessary only if you feel severe pain when you walk. Casting is usually not necessary. However, you will need an orthotic to redistribute your weight so that the bone doesn't crack again when you return to play. Early use of an orthotic will give you relief while the fracture heals.

A stress fracture of the fifth metatarsal, behind the little toe, is a more serious injury. This results from an excessive load on the outside of the foot, such as with the supinating foot. These fractures heal poorly and require early medical attention. Simple rest is not the answer. You may be in a cast and on crutches for anywhere from 6 weeks to several months. Many of these fractures are treated surgically, with a screw used to hold the fragments together.

To avoid getting a stress fracture, wear a shock-absorbing shoe with a good arch and do flexibility and strengthening exercises for the feet, ankles, and legs.

✚ TOE TENDINITIS

Tenderness and swelling along the top of the foot *only* is usually due to tendinitis, an inflammation of the tendons that raise the toes. It will hurt if you hold your toes down with your fingers and try to pull them back up against resistance.

The cause may simply be that you are lacing your shoes too tightly. Or you may have poor padding under the tongues of your tennis shoes.

The treatment is to ice the tendon intermittently until the pain and swelling subside and to take anti-inflammatory agents. I also suggest that you go to an upholstery store and get a wad of foam to put under the tongues of your shoes.

✚ BLISTERS

Blisters form from an improperly fitting tennis shoe. New shoes should be broken in by wearing them around the house.

To treat a blister, open it at the top with a sterilized, sharp instrument, but leave the covering intact. Cover the blister with an antibiotic and a dressing. Blister-prone tennis players can use insoles to reduce friction, wear extra cotton or polypropelene socks, lubricate the foot with Vaseline, or apply tape or moleskin to cover pressure points on the foot.

✚ ATHLETE'S FOOT

Tennis tends to be a sweaty game, and therefore tennis players' shoes and feet can become soaked with sweat. Hot, sweaty feet provide a good breeding ground for fungal infections. Itching and cracking between the toes due to a fungus is called athlete's foot. It can be treated with an antifungal cream or spray available in a drugstore. If athlete's foot persists, see a doctor to obtain a prescription for a stronger antifungal agent.

If you are prone to athlete's foot, make sure the upper of your tennis shoe is made of a breathable material; look for mesh or air vents. Wash and dry your feet immediately after a match or practice, taking care to dry between the toes. If you're changing in a locker room, put on a clean pair of socks; don't wear the sweaty ones home. Don't walk around barefoot in the locker room, where you place yourself at risk of picking up fungal infections. Wear rubber flip-flops back and forth to the shower.

TENNIS SHOE DERMATITIS

Rashes of the feet are often attributed to athlete's foot, but now doctors warn that not all rashes of the feet are fungal in origin. Many wearers of tennis shoes suffer from a contact dermatitis caused by a skin reaction to chemicals used in the manufacture of the shoes. An area of particular concern are the components of the rubber insoles of many of these shoes.

The problem is exacerbated for tennis players when their increased activity causes sweating of the feet, which brings the chemicals from the insole into contact with the foot. The only solution to the problem is to eliminate the contact, which in the case of tennis shoes is virtually impossible. Skin tests can diagnose contact dermatitis, but 20 to 30 percent of people with so-called tennis shoe dermatitis do not test positive. If you have this condition, keep your feet dry as much as possible. Some doctors prescribe corticosteroid lotions and creams for mild cases, but these may become ineffective over time.

CHOOSING A TENNIS SHOE

A tennis player's shoes are an essential part of the equipment. Like other areas of tennis equipment, tennis shoe design has become a high-tech specialty. Dozens of new shoes are introduced each year; some are lighter, others are heavier. The latest trend incorporates a technology that keeps your feet lower to the ground so that the shoes strike the ground at the same points as your feet, which enhances speed and stability.

By wearing proper tennis shoes, you can reduce the risk of all the injuries that stem from a poor foot strike and lead to pain all the way up the leg to the back. You should be able to find a good pair of tennis shoes for between $60 and $80.

Tennis shoes should provide good lateral support and good shock absorption. They should be sturdy and strong with flat soles and a hard, squared-off edge. Also look for a reinforced front, a cushioned midsole, a firm, well-padded heel counter, and a sole with circles to facilitate turning. If your ankles roll over easily, consider heavier, more supportive shoes with a guarantee on the outsole.

Replace worn-out tennis shoes. Patches or other repairs are only temporary fixes, at best, and excessively worn shoes can affect both your feet and your playing style.

When buying new shoes, practice some on-court moves at the store to make sure the shoes fit and feel comfortable. Wait until the afternoon when your feet are going through their midday swell. The shoes should feel comfortable from the moment you try them on; you should not have to break in tennis shoes.

Socks have improved as well. Try tennis socks made of acrylic, not cotton, that wick away perspiration and reduce friction. While cotton absorbs perspiration, it doesn't evaporate it. Reduced friction can help you avoid blisters.

Part Four

Tennis for Everyone

The Senior Game
Women in Tennis
The Junior Player

16

The Senior Game

Molly, an 83-year-old tennis player, came to me because her elbow was bothering her. She played tennis every afternoon with her girlfriends, and she had begun to feel pain right after playing. I put Molly on a light weight-training program using dumbbells and stretching, and I told her to come back in a few weeks. When she returned, she said her elbow hurt even more. So I sat her down and had her describe her rehabilitation program to find out exactly what she was doing. Rather than doing 50 repetitions of the exercises I had given her, she was doing 500. No wonder her elbow pain was worse! I found it hard to yell at a well-meaning Jewish grandmother, so I asked her granddaughter to make sure Molly did only as much as she was supposed to do, not 10 times more. Within a few months, Molly was again playing pain-free on the tennis court.

There is a common misconception that older people should remain sedentary because exercise could cause injuries and place undue strain on the heart. However, research now shows that much of what doctors have ascribed to aging is actually due to inactivity. Exercise is good for people regardless of their age. The United States Tennis Association certainly agrees: it starts senior players at age 45 and increases age brackets by 5 years all the way up to age 85.

Some doctors flatly state that anyone over 35 or 40 should check with a doctor before beginning a new exercise program or taking up a sport like tennis. I don't agree. If you have been exercising regularly for many years, you probably can continue to exercise quite safely without a doctor's prescription. Only those people with known chronic diseases, such as high blood pressure, heart disease, lung disease, and diabetes, need to consult a doctor first.

Someone who decides late in life to take up tennis needs to avoid undue stress on the heart. A sedentary older person who decides to start exercising regularly should have a complete, thorough checkup, particularly to ascertain the status of the heart. Singles tennis involves bursts of activity, and can have serious consequences if your heart is not up to it.

This does not mean that if you have heart disease you can't play tennis. Tennis will benefit someone with mild to moderate heart disease by strengthening the entire cardiovascular system. Your doctor can set limits and outline appropriate levels of playing. You should start playing at a low level and advance very slowly so that you don't overstress your body.

WHAT WE LOSE WITH AGE

Overuse injuries in older tennis players are more likely to have physical consequences than similar injuries in younger players. The treatment of the older player is complicated by the fact that age-related changes may occur in the joints, muscles, bones, ligaments, cartilage, tendons, and joint fluid.

Tennis players who play regularly seem to maintain their abilities better than those who play only intermittently. However, all of us lose quickness, muscle strength, and flexibility as we age.

Quickness is reflected in both the ability to move from one point on the court to another and the ability to bring the racquet rapidly into position. Lower-body quickness seems to diminish more rapidly than upper-body quickness: the old adage that it's the legs that go first seems to be true for aging tennis players. However, experience and anticipation can help you make up for losing a step or two.

Lower-body strength is vital for maintaining speed on the court. Good upper-body strength translates into racquet speed, which is a major factor in how hard you hit the ball. It also helps prevent rotator cuff injuries and tennis elbow.

In the upper body, a loss of flexibility in the shoulder decreases the arc of the serving motion, which decreases racquet speed. In the lower body, this loss shortens your stride, which affects foot speed. Less flexible calf muscles can lead to muscle tears and Achilles tendon rupture.

MIDDLE-AGED ATHLETES

Since the 1970s, many more members of the baby boom generation have been working out and playing lifetime sports such as tennis. Athletes in their 40s and 50s should continue to exercise at whatever level they are capable of. They should not feel that because they are over 40 they have to cut back. In fact, the Nuveen Tour for those 35 and up shows that even aging tennis stars like Jimmy Connors and John McEnroe can still compete at a high level.

If you are playing tennis at a competitive level at age 39 or 49, the change in your game at age 40 or 50 should be totally insignificant. Keep doing what you have been doing until, for some reason, you can't do it any more. However, with increasing age, it becomes more and more important to listen to your body. It will tell you when you are abusing it and when you should begin to back off. Injury or sickness can also cause a tennis player to reduce his or her playing time.

Although players of almost any age may become injured, a handful of tennis injuries are more prevalent among those in their 40s and 50s, including knee cartilage tears, tennis leg, Achilles tendon rupture, tennis elbow, and rotator cuff tendinitis.

Knee Cartilage Tears

Tennis-related knee cartilage tears usually occur in players over age 45, and particularly among those who play intensely. The basic problem is that the aging knee cartilage loses some of its water content and elasticity and, consequently, some internal strength. These changes make tears more likely.

Tears occur when the player lands, anchors the foot, and then attempts an inward or outward pivoting motion. Most players experience some pain and may feel tearing within the knee, although some feel no tearing and have relatively little, if any, pain. A swollen knee on the day following a painful episode is a good indication that damage has occurred. Medial cartilage tears (on the inside of the knee) are more common than lateral cartilage tears (on the outside of the knee).

Many tennis players simply live with a cartilage tear that does not bother them too much. Even a highly active player, who is much more likely to have symptoms, may only feel intermittent pain.

If a cartilage tear remains painful even after conservative treatment (use of anti-inflammatory agents, decreased activity, and quadriceps-strengthening exercises; see pages 28 and 124), then arthroscopic surgery can remove the torn portion. This should be followed by rehabilitation of the leg muscles to help regain full range of motion.

Most tennis players who have torn cartilage can return to play at the same level, even if they need surgery more than once for tearing knee cartilage.

Tennis Leg

Tennis leg is an injury of aging players, and usually occurs while the player is pushing off to rush the net after a serve. Some players feel tightness or cramping in the gastrocnemius muscle behind the lower leg for several weeks beforehand. Then they feel the "pop" of the plantaris tendon, which is similar to the experience of a rupturing Achilles tendon, but higher in the calf.

Immediate compression from the toes to the knee, icing, and elevation help decrease swelling in the leg. Most patients find that they can walk unaided with a flat-footed gait, but some may prefer to use crutches. I encourage a return to normal gait as quickly as possible, realizing that the toe push-off will be difficult at first.

Patients with a more complete tendon rupture may find that walking with the heel elevated makes for a smoother and less painful gait. They must, however, continue to do stretching exercises (Wall Push-ups, and Heel Drops, page 13) to prevent tightening of the gastrocnemius and the Achilles tendon. You must stretch both the injured and the uninjured gastrocnemius muscle and Achilles tendon, since there is a slight chance that this injury will occur on the uninvolved side. When you can stretch the injured calf as far as the normal one without pain, usually within two to three weeks, you can return to playing tennis.

Achilles Tendon Rupture

A total rupture of the Achilles tendon is more of a problem than tennis leg. This injury again occurs during a serve, especially when running in.

Although young players may experience an Achilles tendon rupture, it is typically an injury of those in the 35- to 55-year-old group. Tendons become weaker and less elastic with age.

You will feel a popping sensation with sudden pain that usually relents within a few minutes. You may be able to walk flat-footed, but generally it's impossible to rise up on your tiptoes or run, which is convincing evidence to stop playing.

This is a serious injury. It requires surgical repair of the Achilles tendon, followed by a prolonged rehabilitation program (see page 138). This should bring you back to full physical activity and functional strength.

Tennis Elbow

While hitting a backhand well generally helps prevent tennis elbow, you may still develop this condition if you hit enough backhands within a short period. The majority of those afflicted with tennis elbow are over age 35. This reflects an age-related change in the connective tissue in the arm and elbow.

The hallmarks of tennis elbow are elbow tenderness and pain when hitting the ball and when trying to grip the racquet. The onset of pain is usually insidious, but may occur suddenly, particularly when you have played a great deal of tennis over a short period, switched to a new racquet or new stringing, or played on a hard surface against a hard hitter.

The treatment of tennis elbow depends, to a certain extent, on its severity. Some players have minimal pain and are able to continue playing. They may be helped by using a counterforce brace. Players with more severe pain need to stop playing temporarily and begin a program of gradual resistance exercises to strengthen the wrist and forearm muscles (see pages 99 to 102).

Rotator Cuff Tendinitis

As with tennis elbow, rotator cuff tendinitis usually occurs in those over age 35, although this is also the most common tennis injury among teenage tennis players. The service motion is usually responsible for rotator cuff damage. While it is possible for one violent overhead shot or one serve to produce such an injury, it is unlikely. More commonly, rotator cuff tendinitis occurs insidiously, with gradual increase in pain.

Players usually complain of pain when the arm is raised overhead. The pain worsens with playing, and frequently persists after the game is over, sometimes even into the night. Sleeping is difficult because you may roll over on the injured shoulder, causing severe pain.

I used to tell players with rotator cuff tendinitis that they could continue to hit ground strokes but should stop hitting serves and overheads temporarily. Recent research, however, has revealed that one of the rotator cuff muscles is active throughout the backhand and forehand strokes as well. So it would be wise for an older player to avoid hitting the ball completely while the shoulder is still sore.

Although you must rest, you should maintain full range of motion in the injured shoulder. Work hard on strengthening the rotator cuff muscles, following a shoulder rehabilitation program (see page 78).

Among older players, chronic tendinitis may proceed to rupture of the rotator cuff, which is not usually seen among younger players. So make sure to rehabilitate the shoulder properly before going out to play again, or you may need surgery to repair the tear.

ELDERLY PLAYERS

Elderly players are capable of participating in tennis just as easily as younger ones do. But they do need to take care to warm up properly. The warm-up and warm-down periods should be almost as long as the exercise session itself. Take 10 to 20 minutes to warm up, then exercise for 20 to 30 minutes, and take another 10 to 20 minutes to warm down.

Once you have warmed up, stretch, and then do a tennis warm-up. Bounce a ball off the racquet for a minute or two. Volley back and forth standing in place close to the net. Have a leisurely rally for several minutes at the baseline, avoiding lunges or extreme motions.

An older tennis player's injuries may take longer to heal, so be careful to rehabilitate yourself fully, and slowly, before returning to activity. Also, a senior player is much more likely to suffer from heat stress and dehydration than a younger one. So make sure to drink plenty of liquids before and during playing tennis.

Alternate days of intense activity with light activity. Older tissues need at least 24 hours to recover, so don't play tennis two days in a row. Do light exercise or a different activity on alternate days.

The Benefits of Exercise

The growing number of senior tennis players reflects people's desire for physical fitness and a sense of well-being. The role of regular exercise, such as playing tennis three times a week, in preventing and treating illnesses is well documented, and senior players are increasingly aware of these benefits and are motivated to continue playing tennis.

Exercise strengthens the heart and lungs, lowers blood pressure and cholesterol, thickens bones, tones muscles, and may improve memory. Moderate exercise, such as doubles tennis, also seems to boost the immune system and improve the reflexes of senior players. Because of these benefits, senior tennis players who exercise tend to outlive their inactive contemporaries by two or three years. Even if they don't live longer, they will probably live better and remain independent longer. Thus, exercise improves the quality as well as the quantity of life.

Arthritis

Osteoarthritis is a wear-and-tear phenomenon in which the joint cartilage begins to succumb to overuse. In tennis, the most commonly affected joints are the knees and the hips. Persistent pain in either joint should lead to a doctor's examination and an X ray.

Whether you have played tennis for years or are interested in taking up the game at a later age, arthritis does not have to slow you down. Tennis can be tailored to meet the physical capabilities of almost anyone. If you have arthritis, playing tennis can keep your trunk, hips, and shoulders mobile, plus help you maintain handgrip strength.

Arthritis patients need to learn to modify their equipment to fit their medical condition. Grips, racquets, braces, and shoes can be adapted to fit your needs and abilities. Your local pro shop or tennis specialty store can help you select products to make tennis easier on your joints.

Here are some recommended guidelines to follow:

- Use lightweight racquets to help absorb shock better. The new generation of ultralight, jumbo racquets are aimed specifically at older players. Try an extra-long racquet for more power with less effort.
- Build up the grip size on your racquet with tape or add on a second grip to help you hold the racquet more easily and to reduce stress and pain on your finger joints.
- Try wearing wrist braces and gloves on your racquet hand to stabilize your joints.
- Wear comfortable, lightweight tennis shoes.

A good conditioning program is essential for all tennis players, but especially if your joints need extra protection. Proper conditioning helps maintain range of motion in the joints and reduces your chances of injury.

When you take lessons, don't be afraid to explain your physical limitations to your teaching pro. If you don't have a teaching pro, your local tennis club or tennis specialty shop should be able to recommend someone who assists people with physical limitations.

If you are looking for something to do with your old tennis balls, how about turning them into exercise equipment? A tennis ball, even an old one, is virtually impossible to squeeze with one hand. But you can reduce the ball's resistance by cutting a slit, from 1 inch to 3 inches, into the ball with a knife. Or cut a ball in half for even less resistance.

Using balls with three different resistance levels can help an arthritis patient increase forearm and hand strength. Start with 10 repetitions at the easiest resistance and increase to the next level when that feels comfortable.

Once you are on the court, there are other adaptations that can make the game more enjoyable and safer for your joints:

- Always loosen up beforehand with a proper warm-up and stretching. Spend 10 to 15 minutes warming up; easy practice swings, trunk twists, and walking are good warm-up exercises. Then hit 10 to 15 forehands and 10 to 15 backhands and ease your way into volleys and serves.

- Keep your grip tension on the club consistent to add consistency to your swing and to heighten your overall comfort.

- Listen to your body throughout the game. If you begin to tire, simply end the match, postpone finishing it, or practice hitting ground strokes.

Joint Replacement

Arthritis can cause joints to deteriorate to the point where they need replacing. But there is no reason for a joint replacement to prevent a full return to tennis. Even people who have two artificial hip prostheses can continue to play doubles. One caveat is to avoid playing in wet weather, which increases your chances of slipping and falling.

17

Women in Tennis

In the mid-1980s during the Mahwah Invitational Tournament in New Jersey, Martina Navratilova used to work out at my training facility, the Fitness and Back Institute in Paramus. Watching her work out, it was easy to see why she so dominated women's tennis. In all my years as a sports doctor, I've never seen a female athlete work at such an intensity level. She would do strength training for several hours each day she didn't play tennis. I was totally impressed with the massive number of repetitions and the total amount of weight she lifted, particularly in working the upper body.

A woman's tennis injuries are basically the same as a young man's, but there are some peculiarities due to differences in anatomy, including problems related to the menstrual cycle, growth spurts, and aging bones. The female player also has different nutritional needs than a male player.

SHOULDER PROBLEMS

The repetitive overhead motions of tennis (serve, overheads) cause the rotator cuff muscles in the shoulder to stretch out and become lax. The weaker these muscles are, the more quickly laxity sets in. This results in an impingement of the two biceps tendons in the shoulder. The impingement causes inflammation and shoulder pain that limits your ability to play.

So it's important for women to work hard to build up the shoulder with an off-court strengthening program. Use the same exercises devised to treat shoulder problems beforehand to prevent them from occurring (see page 78).

RUNNER'S KNEE

Runner's knee is much more common among women than men because a woman's pelvis is wider, making the angle between the thigh and the calf sharper. This increases the tendency for the kneecap to pull out of line and rub on the side of its groove, causing knee pain (see page 127). While the main cause of runner's knee is an abnormal foot strike, a woman tennis player's wider pelvis magnifies the abnormality enough so that she feels the symptoms more severely than a man would.

You feel the pain behind the kneecap or in the back of the knee. Playing tennis makes it worse, but so does sitting with the knee bent for any length of time—for example, while watching a long movie.

You can't change the angle in the knee, so the treatment is to correct the foot strike with an arch support or, in more severe cases, with a custom-made orthotic. Also strengthen your quadriceps muscles in the front of the thigh using the 30° Leg Extension exercise (see page 129).

TENNIS ELBOW

Tennis elbow is usually associated with lack of forearm strength. I see it particularly among women who play mixed doubles. When the ball comes at a woman with more force than she is used to, the shock of the hall hitting the racquet is transmitted up through her forearm. Since the ball is coming so fast, her weight is typically back and she is late getting her racquet head around. On the backhand, if the ball hits the racquet while the elbow is still bent, the shock is transmitted to the outer area of the elbow, causing elbow pain.

Treatment is to ice the elbow and take anti-inflammatories to ease the pain, and then strengthen the muscles in the forearm and wrist (see pages 99 to 102).

KNEE LIGAMENT INJURIES

Recent research shows that women are more likely than men to injure the anterior cruciate ligament (ACL) in the knee, one of the most important ligaments for stabilizing the knee. The ACL is torn more frequently in sports that combine running with sudden direction changes, which includes tennis.

No one knows exactly why women are more susceptible to these injuries, but it may be due to anatomy or differences in muscle strength. The most plausible explanation is that women may have less room than men in the center of the knee. Women with narrow spaces have a higher incidence of ACL injuries because the ACL is more likely to tear in a narrow space.

An ACL injury varies in severity from a mild sprain to a complete ligament tear. A sprain will cause sudden pain and rapid swelling. A complete rupture will cause a loud pop that can be heard by everyone on the court. The knee may feel unstable and have a tendency to collapse if you try to walk.

Both a ligament sprain and a tear should be seen and treated by a physician. A complete tear can often be diagnosed by a physical exam or, if necessary, an MRI scan.

A mild sprain can be treated with ice, anti-inflammatories, and a knee-strengthening program (see page 123). A complete tear requires surgical repair and a six- to nine-month rehabilitation program. In older women tennis players, a good rehabilitation program and knee bracing often will suffice, particularly if they play recreational and not competitive tennis.

Jump training may help you prevent a knee ligament injury. Most serious knee injuries do not involve contact with another player, but occur when you land from a jump. There is a marked imbalance between hamstring muscle and quadriceps muscle strength in female athletes. Also, men tend to use their knee flexor muscles more than women do, which protects the ACL from injury during landing.

A proper jumping technique may help reduce these injuries. Maintain correct posture and body alignment during the jump. Jump straight up and down with no excessive side-to-side or forward-backward motion. Land softly on bent knees, and recoil instantly to prepare for the next stroke. Female players who concentrate on using the proper technique can build a base of strength, power, and agility.

ACHILLES TENDON INJURIES

Women are also subject to a higher incidence of Achilles tendon inflammation or injury. This is not due to innate structural differences, but to prolonged wearing of high heels. Over time, this causes the Achilles tendon to shorten. When it suddenly stretches, by running or lunging for a ball, the tendon may become inflamed or even tear.

Tennis shoes further aggravate the problem: the shoe generally has a flat heel, not the built-up heel of a running shoe. Women's feet are different than men's. Women need shoes with narrower heels, higher arches, and wider toe boxes. New tennis shoes designed specifically for women are now available. These comfortable, lightweight shoes have a shoe last made for a woman, not a scaled-down version of a man's shoe. They come in various width options, mid- and low-cut versions, and with a front that flexes properly in the ball of the foot.

An active stretching program both off the court and before playing will lengthen the Achilles tendon and prevent injury. Do Wall Push-ups and Heel Drops (see page 13).

MENSTRUAL IRREGULARITIES

A major problem among women who are ultraslim and who exercise heavily is amenorrhea, or disruption of the normal menstrual cycle. I see this among young, competitive tennis players.

Intensive physical activity before puberty can delay a girl's first period by a year or more and lead to an irregular menstrual cycle. Numerous theories have been advanced to explain the relationship between exercise and amenorrhea. There seems to be a change in the control of the pituitary and the ovaries, resulting in a dramatic fall in estrogen levels.

A very thin woman with little body fat may experience a hormone imbalance. To maintain the natural rise and fall of hormones during the menstrual cycle, a woman must maintain a body fat content of about 22 percent. Too much exercise along with a rigorous diet may reduce a woman's body fat and cause ovulation problems. Women tennis players with a body fat content of 17 percent or less will not menstruate.

The good news is that this exercise-induced fertility problem appears to be reversible. As soon as you cut down on exercise and gain a few pounds, your body fat will build up again and your period will return to normal. If it doesn't, you should see a gynecologist. You may have other medical problems that need attention.

BONE LOSS AND STRESS FRACTURES

Bone strength is important for women, particularly as they age. A menstrual disturbance in a young female tennis player can increase her risk of bone loss and stress fractures. Amenorrhea, the lack of a menstrual period, in a young player usually leads to insufficient bone mineral density. With aging, she will lose bone tissue and be vulnerable to the bone-wasting disease of osteoporosis.

Osteoporosis is the thinning of the bones due to loss of bone mass. The bones of the skeleton become porous, brittle, and more easily break-able in women and men with osteoporosis. During childhood and early adult life, more bone is made than is broken down. However, by age 35, there is a net loss of bone, which is accelerated around age 65. Osteoporosis affects 25 percent of American women and it may be severe, resulting in crippling and disfigurement. It has been estimated that 1.3 million women per year will have bone fractures because of underlying osteoporosis.

The preponderance of osteoporosis in women is believed to be related to sudden decreases in estrogen levels in their bodies. Estrogen is vital to proper bone growth because it allows calcium to be absorbed from the intestines, and calcium is a necessary ingredient in building the skeleton.

Osteoporosis may become a factor in tennis players due to stress on the spine. A good weight-training program helps to slow the development and degree of osteoporosis. Both estrogen and calcium supplements can help optimize bone mass, but estrogen therapy is controversial. See your doctor for an individual assessment.

Preventing Osteoporosis

There are several factors that may prevent the development of osteoporosis. The first is to take an adequate amount of calcium in the diet throughout life so that bones are built up before bone loss begins at age 35. Estrogen therapy can sometimes be successful, and exercise is beneficial by strengthening the bones.

Diet is extremely important in preventing osteoporosis, and calcium-rich dairy products should be included in the diet. These foods tend to be high in calories and cholesterol, so choose low-fat versions whenever possible. In addition, excessive calcium loss may occur from soft drinks, coffee, alcohol, and nicotine in cigarettes, so limit your intake of these beverages and, of course, try to cut down or stop smoking.

The recommended daily allowance of calcium is 1 gram (1,000 milligrams) for women over age 19 and 1.2 to 1.5 grams (1,200–1,500 milligrams) for women after menopause to avoid osteoporosis. To take in this amount of calcium usually requires calcium supplements since the average American diet contains about 600 or 700 milligrams of calcium.

If you are considering calcium supplements, check with your physician to find the right kind for you.

Several new drugs have won approval from the Food and Drug Administration (FDA) to prevent osteoporosis and fractures in postmenopausal women with osteoporosis, one of the few instances drugs have been indicated to prevent a chronic disease. These new drugs, known as bisphosphonates, including alendronate and etidronate, provide a nonhormonal option for preventing rapid bone loss in the early postmenopausal period, the bone loss that may lead to osteoporosis and fractures.

Weight-bearing exercise, such as tennis, is particularly valuable in reducing bone loss in middle-aged and postmenopausal women. I recommend that all female players get regular, weight-bearing exercise to help prevent osteoporosis.

SPECIAL PROTECTION AND PRECAUTIONS

Upper-Body Strength

Women can build their legs to be extremely strong, but they cannot, in general, develop their upper-body strength as much as men because of basic physiologic differences. The human male has an innate potential to develop bigger shoulders, chest, and arms than the human female.

Through weight training, women can increase their upper-body strength markedly without bulking up as men do. This is because women have little circulating male hormone, which is required for bulking up. The huge upper bodies you see on female weight trainers are due to steroid use. As long as a female tennis player has a normal level of circulating female hormones and doesn't take any artificial male hormones, she will increase her strength and not her bulk through weight training.

Good Nutrition

For general nutritional guidelines, see chapter 2, "Eat to Compete." In addition to those guidelines, women may need to supplement their diets for peak athletic performance. Most women need a high calcium intake. Dairy foods such as low-fat milk, calcium pills, or even a few Tums (which have a high calcium content) a day should provide the calcium a woman needs.

A female needs a higher concentration of iron in her diet than a male, and this is especially true for tennis players. A heavily exercising female player breaks down blood cells at a higher rate than a sedentary woman. This, combined with loss of blood during the menstrual cycle, requires increased intake of iron. I recommend that female tennis players take in 15 milligrams of iron per day, either through the diet or supplements.

Some women are still resistant to a high-carbohydrate diet. The idea that a high-starch diet can be nonfattening is hard for some women to comprehend. Traditionally, when women attempted to diet, they gave up bread, potatoes, and rice. These old dietary prejudices may be hard to overcome.

Protecting the Breasts

Any woman must be concerned with protecting her breasts during sports. Sports bras now provide much-needed breast support. The first sports bra was made in the mid-1970s by sewing two jock straps together. Since then, the market has been flooded with sports bras of different shapes and sizes.

Sports bras are designed to minimize breast motion. They either compress the breasts against the chest or cradle and restrain each breast separately within a cup. There are sports bras for every body style. The ones that press the breasts flat to the chest work well for small- or medium-chested women; those that cup the breasts separately like traditional bras provide good motion control for larger-breasted women.

A good sports bra is sturdy but not constricting and allows a full range of motion. Most are made of nonabrasive, breathable materials. Sweating increases friction, so make sure that the bra has good ventilation and that you shower and dry off immediately after playing tennis.

Since there are so many sports bras available, evaluate each one before you make a purchase. When trying on a bra, run in place or do jumping jacks, and make the motions of a tennis swing. You want to make sure you get all the support you need. The bra should be comfortable every time you put it on and easy to get in and out of. There should be no tenderness or soreness around the rib band under the breasts and no red marks when you take the bra off.

Generally, the wider the back, the more support you have. The shoulder straps should be adjustable and wider than normal straps. Armholes should allow for ample movement. Make sure that hooks or fasteners don't come in contact with the skin.

Practice wear for women now often includes a form-fitting bra top, allowing freedom of movement, along with the latest in breathable material.

Pregnancy Care

Most women can continue to exercise while pregnant. Several world-class tennis players, including Evonne Goolagong, have given birth to healthy babies and gone right back to competing. A pregnant tennis player simply needs to consult her doctor, follow some simple guidelines, and pay attention to her body for signs of fatigue.

In 1994 the American College of Obstetrics and Gynecology (ACOG) revised its guidelines for women who plan to exercise during pregnancy, allowing for greater exercise intensity. These guidelines recommend a target heart rate during pregnancy that is 25 to 30 percent lower than the nonpregnant target. You need to find your own comfortable exercise level. For a fit woman, 30 minutes is probably safe because the blood flow to the uterus is not significantly reduced within this time.

Tennis-playing women certainly shouldn't take nine months off. If a woman is planning a pregnancy, she should exercise to get in shape before she becomes pregnant and then maintain her fitness during pregnancy. Tennis is considered a safe sport during pregnancy, although the risk of sprains may be greater with sudden stops, starts, and changes of direction on the court.

If you do play while pregnant, make sure to drink adequate fluids, up to 1 pint before playing and 1 cup every 20 minutes during the game. Even if you are not thirsty after playing, drink enough to replenish lost fluids. You can lose 1 to 2 liters of fluid per hour through sweating.

Pregnant women also should take care not to play when the weather is hot and humid. In general, the higher the air temperature, the lower the humidity must be to avoid heat problems. For example, if the air temperature is above 80°F, the humidity should be no higher than 50 percent. Also, it's safer to play before 8 A.M. and after 6 P.M.

Water retention in the third trimester may reduce mobility at the wrists and ankles, and lead to carpal tunnel syndrome, causing muscle weakness and pain in the wrists. Activities such as tennis, which require strength and agility of the hands, may make pregnant women more injury-prone.

Exercising after Birth

Fit women tend to rebound quickly from childbirth. Most postpartum classes offer strength-training routines and exercises similar to those of prenatal classes. These classes help women build strength in the abdominal, back, and shoulder muscles, which is necessary for hoisting a baby around. Playing tennis can help a woman shed the extra pounds gained during pregnancy. Within a month of giving birth, a woman should be able to see improvements in her aerobic capacity.

Many women who breast-feed are fearful that exercise may hinder their milk supply. But active women actually produce more milk than inactive women.

Before a woman starts a postpartum workout, she should check with her doctor.

Relieving Menstrual Woes

A regular game of tennis may help relieve the painful, disabling symptoms of premenstrual syndrome as well as those of menopause. Exercise causes the pituitary gland to release endorphins, a group of substances chemically similar to morphine and thought to be the source of the elusive runner's high. Studies show that exercise can help ameliorate the aches and abdominal cramps associated with menstrual changes.

SPECIAL BENEFITS FOR WOMEN WHO EXERCISE

Exercise may benefit women even more than men. Running around the tennis court helps to reduce bone loss and prevent osteoporosis. Bone densities are much higher in exercising women than in those who are sedentary.

Also, women who exercise regularly starting at a young age are less likely to develop breast cancer. Obesity increases the risks of breast cancer, and exercise helps women remain lean. Researchers have reported lower rates of breast and reproductive system cancers in women who were athletes in college compared to their nonactive classmates.

In addition, elderly women who regularly perform endurance exercises have been found to undergo greater changes in cholesterol level compared with middle-aged women who exercise.

18

The Junior Player

Within the last decade or so, the highest ranking professional tennis players have become younger and younger. This tendency applies to both men and women players, although the younger generation of women, led by Martina Hingis, Venus Williams, and Anna Kournikova, now seems to dominate the women's game. The top men's players seem to mature somewhat later, partly because they are still getting stronger into their 20s, and strength is an integral part of tennis. Also, girls tend to mature physiologically earlier than boys.

Nowadays, many players turn professional between the ages of 15 and 17. They start full-time practice at much earlier ages because of the technical complexity of tennis and the high degree of motor skills required. The best time to acquire these skills has been shown to be between ages 10 and 12 for girls and ages 10 and 13 for boys. During this period, the differences between boys and girls in the development of their performance are very small; therefore, professional practice is begun during childhood.

Unfortunately, this heavy load of training can lead to acute and overuse injuries. A junior tennis player's parents, coach, and physician all need to monitor how a young athlete's growing body reacts to high amounts of practice time. In addition to the typical ills and injuries associated with tennis, such as knee ligament injuries, dislocated kneecap, runner's knee, shoulder impingement, tennis elbow, and cracked vertebrae in the back, younger players have a special set of problems, including growth-plate injuries in the bones.

KNEE LIGAMENT INJURIES

Female tennis players, including young ones, have an increased incidence of sprains and ruptures of the anterior cruciate ligament (ACL) in the knee, one of the knee's most crucial supporting structures. When you plant your foot and rotate your knee, you can stretch the ACL. For a very mild sprain, the immediate treatment is to use the RICE formula (see page 46) and then do leg-strengthening exercises such as the Leg Extension (see page 27) and the Leg Curl (see page 28). A moderate or severe sprain should be looked at by a doctor.

An ACL rupture, which causes a loud pop, sudden pain, and instability of the knee, is a much more severe injury. An MRI scan can tell whether the ligament is partially or totally torn. A partial tear can be rehabilitated with the aid of a physical therapist. A total tear requires surgical repair with a recovery time of six to seven months after a laborious rehabilitation.

DISLOCATED KNEECAP

Dislocated kneecaps are particularly prevalent among tennis players because of the sudden changes in direction the game demands. This injury is also more common among teenage female players compared to teenage male players. The groove that the kneecap rides in is generally much shallower in women than in men. In teenage girls, the outer rim of the groove is still underdeveloped, allowing the kneecap to slide to the outside as the knee twists. The kneecap therefore has less lateral stability.

If the kneecap slides partially out and snaps back in, this is a partial dislocation, or subluxation. You will feel sudden pain with tenderness in the knee and have some swelling. See a doctor to determine the extent of the damage to the tissues that hold the kneecap in place. Apply ice to keep the swelling down. A knee immobilizer will stabilize the kneecap and allow the damaged tissues to heal. It usually takes 10 to 14 days to heal.

If the kneecap slides all of the way out and stays out, this is a total dislocation. The kneecap will sit on the outer side of the knee. A doctor can usually put the kneecap back in place fairly easily in young girls because the outer rim of the groove is still underdeveloped. However, in some cases it can be difficult, and may even require anesthesia to put it back in place.

A totally dislocated kneecap requires a more prolonged period of immobilization because of the increased damage. This should be followed by a quadriceps-strengthening program of Leg Extensions (see page 27). In rare instances, surgery may be necessary to stabilize the kneecap.

RUNNER'S KNEE

Runner's knee is much more common among women than men because a woman's pelvis is wider, making the angle between the thigh and the calf sharper. This increases the tendency for the kneecap to pull out of line and rub on the side of its groove, causing knee pain.

A woman player susceptible to this condition may first feel the knee pain as an adolescent. An increase in activity, or playing on hard surfaces for prolonged times, may cause inflammation severe enough to finally cause pain.

Ice and anti-inflammatories can control the pain. Either an inexpensive arch support or, if the pain is quite severe, a more expensive, custom-made orthotic should be enough to allow you to return to playing again.

Adolescent tennis players should also stretch their thigh muscles to reduce the chance of runner's knee pain. Adolescent growth, and especially the growth spurt, can cause a relative period of decreased flexibility. Tennis players with runner's knee who seek attention for their pain often become frustrated when no significant injury is found, and they continue to have pain.

I try to stress the importance of quadriceps stretching (see page 119) to junior players, and have them demonstrate the proper technique for me. Young tennis players who experience continued pain despite improved thigh muscle flexibility must be reevaluated for other potential problems, including local pathology that may require surgery.

SHOULDER IMPINGEMENT

A lack of upper-body strength can cause rotator cuff muscles to become lax and the biceps tendons to become impinged in the shoulder joint. The follow through (deceleration) phase of the serve is the most injurious, as it is in throwing sports.

Young tennis players tend to get loose shoulders that have no symptoms. Rotator cuff tightening through strengthening exercises is important before symptoms appear. In young girls, immaturity is also a factor in decreased muscle development and strength, and they certainly would benefit by exercises to strengthen the rotator cuff muscles (see page 78).

CRACKED BACK

A crack in the vertebrae in the back, known as spondylolysis, is a more common injury in tennis than in many sports kids play. Young tennis players develop these stress fractures because of the recurrent arching of the back during the serving motion. One suspicious sign of this injury is pain on one side of the back that is aggravated by serving.

Treatment involves a prolonged rest period of up to six months to see whether the fracture will heal by itself, followed by a back-strengthening program (see page 91).

TENNIS ELBOW

Tennis elbow occurs often in both female adolescents and adults. The problem usually stems from the shock of hitting the ball, often from a poorly hit backhand stroke, being transmitted up through the forearm.

Another complicating factor involves stress on the growth plate in the elbow of a young player. Constant overuse places stress in the elbow and can widen the growth plate, with subsequent overgrowth of bone on the outside of the elbow.

The treatment is to rest the elbow by not playing tennis. If the pain is not severe, icing the elbow and taking anti-inflammatory agents will allow the young tennis player to continue to play.

If the pain becomes severe, the junior player must cease activity entirely. Some young players hit serves so hard that they tear the knob of bone off the elbow. The bone must then be reattached surgically and the elbow allowed to heal, and the youngster must refrain from playing tennis or throwing altogether.

GROWTH-PLATE INJURIES

Problems can arise when young athletes push themselves to the point of overuse injuries, as often happens with competitive junior players.

The trauma of long-term training can damage joints that aren't completely developed. Before age 13, any activity that requires high-intensity training can affect a child's physical development by putting stress on the growth plates, the growing areas at the ends of bones at the joints. This is less of a problem among older teens, who have gone through most of their growth spurts.

The most common growth-plate injury is Osgood-Schlatter disease, which causes swelling and marked tenderness in a lump of bone just below the knee. This piece of bone is the tibial tubercle, the area where the tendon from the kneecap attaches to the shinbone. It contains a growth center that controls the growth of the tubercle itself, not the whole leg. As the young player gets bigger and heavier, the knob has to become bigger for the attachment of the tendon. In some youngsters, the repetitive yanking of the kneecap tendon as they flex and extend the knee while playing tennis causes the growth center in the tubercle to become irritated. When a growth center is irritated, it becomes painful and is stimulated to overgrow.

Osgood-Schlatter disease, like most growth-plate injuries, is self-limiting; that is, it always goes away by itself. By the time a young tennis player reaches age 17, the growth center closes, and the tendon is then pulling on a solid knob of bone. The pain disappears, but the lump under the knee does not. It is a permanent fixture in the bone.

This disease is self-limiting also because the more it hurts, the harder it is for the child to play tennis. In the past, doctors limited what kids could do, and some kids sat out as much as two years waiting for the growth center to close. There is absolutely no reason for this, and we now allow a child to do whatever he or she can.

Only when the junior player says, "I can't play tennis any more. It hurts too much," do I prescribe a knee immobilizer. The immobilizer keeps the knee straight and prevents the tendon from yanking on the growth center, which relieves the pain. This also prevents the young player from running around, so the pain doesn't recur. The immobilizer is taken off every night to allow the youngster to shower and to test the tibial tubercle. When the bump under the knee is no longer tender to the touch, then he or she can return to activity.

Ice and aspirin or anti-inflammatory agents are also used to relieve any pain. Virtually all junior players can continue to play through this disability.

SPECIAL CONCERNS AND PRECAUTIONS

Pressure to Perform

From age six on up, children are pressured to participate in organized, competitive tennis. Everything today seems to be organized, with weekly junior tournaments and rigidly scheduled leagues. Yet sports competition should be no more or no less stressful than performing in the school play or playing in the school band.

The pressures of organized leagues can be difficult for children. It's not that they don't want to have fun, but that the parents and coaches take the fun out of the game for them. With so much pressure on them to win, they tend to burn out at an early age. Look how long it's taken teenage phenom Jennifer Capriati to get her game back in shape after she burned out.

I see junior tennis players who don't want to play tennis any more. They come into my office with symptoms of injuries or overuse syndromes. They are afraid to tell their coach or their parents that they don't want to play, so they hide behind recurrent injuries. Parents need to be sensitive to the hidden language behind the excuses children use to avoid practice or competition.

Fatigue

Fatigue is a common problem among young tennis players. Teens need sleep to help their bodies grow. They also need extra energy to help their bodies grow, and this comes from a good, healthy diet.

Some teens lack sufficient iron in their bodies. Even though their iron deficiency may not be severe enough to produce anemia, it can slow their growth, deplete their energy supply, and lead to poor sports performance. Although iron deficiency is usually associated with girls, boys also lose iron during strenuous exercise.

In general, I don't think vitamin supplements are appropriate for young tennis players. Most of them eat a lot, and as long as they eat a balanced diet, they don't need vitamin supplements. For a picky eater, supplements may be beneficial.

Sensitivity to Temperature

Young tennis players take longer to adjust to abrupt increases in heat and humidity than older players do. Therefore, they have an increased risk of dehydration in hot weather. Make sure junior players take in enough liquids before, during, and after matches to replenish lost fluids.

A Stretching Program

The physical demands of tennis cause certain adaptations by the young player's body. These adaptations are often positive, such as an increase in muscular strength. However, repeated demands on muscles and tendons may cause a decrease in normal joint range of motion.

Young, competitive tennis players spend the majority of their time playing or practicing tennis, averaging 20 or more hours per week and playing six days per week. These players show a decrease in ability to inwardly rotate both of their shoulder joints, particularly on the dominant side. This can be explained as a muscular adaptation to hitting hundreds of ground strokes. They also have an increase in shoulder external rotation, which is a likely adaptation to the tennis serve. These young players also have a significant reduction in low-back flexibility and have decreased hamstring flexibility.

Tightness in the internal rotation of shoulders of young tennis players can be a source of potential injury and decreased performance. Tight shoulder muscles increase the chances of overload on the shoulder. A flexibility program for tennis should concentrate on improving internal shoulder rotation. Shoulder inflexibility may force the young player to alter his or her form, which may become a factor in elbow injuries. Altering form to overcome shoulder tightness may also reduce the velocity of the serve.

Lower-back pain is a common complaint among elite tennis players. The ballistic nature of tennis and the body position necessary to play the sport are factors that may cause a cycle of lower-back tightness and muscular weakness.

A flexibility program for young tennis players should concentrate on the lower-back area. Inflexibility of the lower back has been shown to be a contributing factor in back pain. By concentrating on lower-back flexibility, the young player can help prevent one of the more common injuries in tennis.

Other areas of the body, including the neck, legs, arms, and wrists, should not be ignored. You should probably spend more time stretching areas you have identified as tight, but do an overall stretching program. Stretching both before and after playing may be ideal, but may not always be practical. Stretch within reason in terms of your time constraints. Try to do a general whole body stretch before playing, followed by a shorter stretching program afterward for your individual tight spots.

Index